REVOLUTION
OF THE SPIRIT
Awaken the Healer

GERRI RAVYN STANFIELD

Revolution of the Spirit: Awaken the Healer
First Edition, Holy Risk Press, June 2016
Copyright © 2016
Gerri Ravyn Stanfield
All rights reserved

Published 2016 by Holy Risk Press

Cover Art and Design:
© 2016 Caitlin Harris

Interior Design and Layout:
© 2016 Diane Rigoli, RigoliCreative.com

Editing:
Jennifer Ruby Privateer
Vanessa Veselka

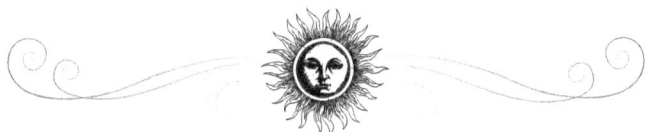

TABLE OF CONTENTS

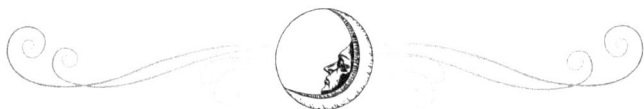

For Momo, who taught me the power of stories.

For all the ones who kept the wonder in medicine, the miracle workers, the healers all over the world who never let the spirit die.

For Lynx, Dawn and Ravenna and your unflinching belief in me.

For all of you who need revolutionary healing the most, I wrote this book for you.

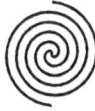

An Open Invitation to Become a Global Revolutionary Healer

"No cure that fails to engage our spirit can make us well."

– Viktor Frankl

In some parallel universe of the great space-time continuum, you and I sit together with a cold summer beer on the porch stoop. Or we prop ourselves up with giant squishy cushions on the coral colored sofa in my living room with a winter cup of tea. You ask me if I believe we can really heal the world, change our industrialized consumer culture into something life-giving. You confess that you struggle to find hope when everything is crumbling around us. You lean over. You want to conspire. You whisper your most pressing, unrelenting desire for all beings to be loved and free, even if it seems impossible.

We pause here and give ourselves the gift of real breath, not the shallow survival chest breath, but the gritty bottomless kind. The breath that unclenches the tight places. The breath that coats our entire insides. Our old friend, oxygen pours into our shapes and changes everything.

During all our profound breathing, I press my hand to my own belly, thanking the divine in the way that I know this ineffable Source. My stomach offers a small burp (remember the beer or tea we just drank), just in case I take myself too damn seriously. The heart flame that dances inside my rib cage meets the privilege that I did not earn from wearing pale skin in the world. I touch your shoulder so you know I am right here.

I tell you that hope is a personal practice, a martial art. There is no guarantee of winning the world that we want and no one knows how anything will go. Ingenious solutions to impossible problems are required daily. All I really understand is that I must dream the beginning of the world instead of the end. Every day. Even when I don't want to. Even when I am crumpled on the floor with my depression or smashing aluminum cans in my recycling bin with my rage.

If you think you know what I mean, I wrote this book for you. Let's spend some time together in the nexus where science and art, medicine and spirituality meet and then, kiss.

We live in interesting times. The modern world is immediate and frequently brutal. Most of us who live in developed countries are not searching for our next meal but we still feel hungry. For some of us, our hunger pushes us to dive into our own soul fire and find the medicine that lives inside of us. There is a service and responsibility asked of you and me, of all of us who have time, passion, energy and resources right now. Our collective work is to stop the damage and restore the spirit of humanity. Or more simply put for the rugged individual, to do the thing you do.

In times of transformation, it is the skills of the healer that need to take center stage. These times cry out for healers who are willing to take holy risks, to develop innovative and unusual plans to treat the modern diagnoses from which our whole planet suffers.

I know there is a kind of medicine that you practice or seek for your own life. If you are doing anything in any community to offer comfort, relief, the potential for change or a more jubilant way of living, you already bring healing. Maybe you have spent years in training to be a doctor or maybe you heal in quiet ways that no one has ever seen before. Maybe something you can't quite name excites or frightens you about being told you have medicine to offer.

There is an acupuncture treatment known as The Seven Dragons. When a person is possessed by demons, needles are inserted at seven points to awaken powerful dragon protectors inside the body to chase the demons away.

My graduate school Chinese Medicine professor taught us this as a treatment for possession in our third year Differential Diagnosis class. We imagined ourselves as the priest in The Exorcist who could cast out demons while Linda Blair spit green pea soup everywhere. We all giggled. My teacher said that possession comes in many forms. In the modern world, it often looks like unremitting depression, obsessive thinking, manic episodes, insomnia, despair, addiction, eating disorders, panic attacks. I understood how all of those conditions manifest like a demon 'possessing' someone, taking over their bodies and lives. I was certain that if I brought it up as an option, my patients would either scream with laughter or back slowly out the door.

My professor declared that our patients would literally ask us for this de-possession treatment. She instructed us to watch for poor eye contact, talk of ghosts and a feeling of absence in the patient's presentation. Look out for strange things for people to do in a doctor's office.

In my third year of practice, a 39 year-old female new patient came in to receive acupuncture for fertility issues. She shredded a tissue in her clenched left hand and kept her eyes on the floorboards. Her tests said not pregnant (again) after sinking thousands of dollars into fertility treatments. I wrote down my usual intake information and then, something inside me pushed me to ask this patient about her dreams. She shuffled her feet from side to side and still did not look at me. "I've been plagued by nightmares where ghosts chase me around, trying to kill me. I'm getting five hours of sleep but it is spread over at least ten hours lying in bed. I just don't feel like myself anymore."

Cultivating fertility is a challenging process with cycles of anticipation and disappointment. When expensive treatments took a long time to produce results, it drained people and left them feeling vulnerable. I imagined that this woman had ridden an emotional roller coaster for a while and might be exhausted. That day, because she showed me all of the odd and very specific 'possession' symptoms, I decided to risk doing something unusual, try the ancient de-possession remedy and see what happened.

"I want to offer something a bit unconventional here. There is a treatment in Chinese Medicine that lifts problems that are weighting us down. Thousands of years ago, it was used to chase away evil spirits, creating doors in the body so protective dragon energies could chase away demons. I find that these days, it helps move the heavy energy of grief, pain, fear and loss so that there is more space for happiness. Fertility is directly affected by our mood and emotions. I would like to start there before we begin to strengthen your reproductive system. Would you be interested in a more extraordinary approach?"

My patient lifted her head an inch higher and showed her face for the first time. "Are you kidding? That is exactly how I have been feeling. Overwhelmed by a weight I can't lift no matter what I do. Let's try it!"

She got on the massage table and we did the Seven Dragons treatment. The tiny, threadlike needles stayed inserted at the seven points for about 45 minutes. All the while, my patient listened to soft music and reclined on the heated table.

She giggled when I removed the acupuncture needles at the end of the treatment. "That was the wildest thing I ever did, I feel so much lighter...even hopeful. This may sound crazy but it felt like something left my body. Wow."

The narrative we know about medicine today is that people get sick, and then visit a health care professional in order to be fixed. Their issues are resolved (or not) and they are sent home or referred to another practitioner.

There is a new kind of sacred medicine for which these times are pleading. In urban culture, we have outbreaks of depression, anxiety and post-traumatic stress. We see rising rates of autoimmune disorders and addiction, along with all the usual challenges the body throws our way. Overuse and exhaustion of the adrenal glands, central to healthy immune system functioning, is another of the latest epidemics. And these are the people who are better off financially and have more access to resources than much of the world's population.

Now is a global moment for healers to offer a different kind of revolutionary leadership to change the consciousness of industrialized culture. We want to touch a larger truth about the repair of the human race and our whole world. We sit beside people and hold their hands in times of personal crisis, to help them see what is next. Our world demands healers to do the same on a wider scale. Healers who are willing to realistically diagnose what is happening and propose unconventional solutions. Right now, healers are required to step out of the treatment room or office and into a global arena where health and justice matters to every single being on our planet.

1. Listen/Ask Questions
2. Diagnose Problem
3. Create Recovery Plan
4. Respond. Reassess

These four steps are foundational to our treatment plans and no less vital to our collective health. Global healers in every culture have utilized these practices for thousands of years. We are now being asked to do the same in contemporary crises. Although swift action is needed in emergencies, healers know how to assess the crisis and determine where it is most effective to respond first. These transformational skills steer us toward the kind of cultural alchemy that we require to survive on our earth.

A fortysomething nurse practitioner in one of my Portland workshops told me that she shies away from the word healer. She said the word suggests that the practitioner does something "to" people. Nothing could be further from the truth. Revolutionary healers invite, and even challenge people toward restoration or complete change. No matter what patients' beliefs are, there is something each person holds sacred that influences their healing process.

We must expand our definition of the word healer to include not only:

- Bodyworkers
- Medical and Natural Physicians
- Caregivers
- Nurses
- Acupuncturists
- Mental Health Therapists
- Physical Therapists
- Occupational and Speech Therapists
- Herbalists
- Energy Workers
- Traditional Shamans/Medicine Workers
- Other physical healing modalities.

But also:

- **Teachers**
- **Inventors**
- **Politicians**
- **Community or movement organizers**
- **Creatrixes**
- **Scientists**
- **Farmers**
- **Consultants**
- **Artists**
- **All the others who are encouraging our modern culture toward wholeness.**

Professors in my graduate school program for acupuncture urged me never to mention spirituality in the treatment room so that patients would take me seriously. I have always been a rule breaker. I am also a spiritual seeker, studying and participating in a multiplicity of services, ceremonies, practices and rituals all over the world. My healing investigations, studies and adventures over the years took me from central Asian shamanic practices, to the earth-based traditions of Northern and Central Europe to the healers of North and South America and the ancient arts of Africa. In my twenties and thirties, I literally went anyplace I was invited to taste the nectar that is our human spirituality and ask people how they healed each other.

My acupuncture patients came with pain in their knees, backs, necks, hips. One came with mind numbing anxiety that would not respond to medication. Another presented with debilitating insomnia that began after a tour in Iraq. Still another came for treatment of unrelenting depression that started six months after his mother died. They came after medication didn't touch it, surgery did not fix it, physical therapy could not restore full function. Multiple doctors told them there was nothing more they could do. Many were suffering, addicted, overworked, jaded and on the verge of hopelessness. They did not leave my office that way.

My own battles with depression, addiction, anxiety and reproductive cancer revealed numerous gaping holes in the opportunities available to those who are desperate to change their lives. If an acupuncturist with years of medical education felt intimidated and discouraged with the current system of health care, how did people who had no training in medicine advocate for themselves?

When all my acupuncture patients independently began to bring up their spiritual crises, I realized that it wasn't just me. We need healers to step forward who are fluent in the language of spirituality. People craved deeper metamorphosis than contemporary medicine often provided. I could embrace the sacred without apology or religious preference and people responded to what they found sacred. When I told my patients or students about my own healing path with cancer, chronic pain or depression, I watched their bodies visibly relax. I knew what it was like to want a miracle.

In the most common forms of Chinese medicine, I would work with my patients to move life force (qi) with hair thin needles inserted into acupuncture points. We treated body and mind, reconnecting sensation and emotion. I introduced enjoyable exercises, personal practices and breath work. As their pain subsided, questions would begin to arise.

Over time, they told me that they needed:

- **Grounding in their physical bodies**
- **Time spent outside or in relaxation**
- **Sacred practices that spoke to their hearts**
- **Integration of their souls into work and relationships**
- **Forgiveness for themselves and others**
- **Grace**
- **Deeper connection with community**
- **Nourishment and change**
- **Confidence in their purpose**
- **Absolute transformation of their lives**

My acupuncture patients did not want excessive talk therapy, organized religion or pop psychology. They wanted hope when medication and surgery were not the only solutions or did not work. They wanted to utterly transmute their patterns and connect with something larger than themselves, something ineffable and real. Many of my patients refused to go back to business as usual. They stopped taking any bullshit in their lives. Our work together created ways to heal their spirit so they could feel free and present with frequent moments of joy.

All true revolutions involve that which is sacred to us. Science now draws the same conclusions that most kinds of human spirituality have taught for thousands of years. We are interconnected, as a human race and as a planet of ecosystems. This underlying unity may be one of the most healing truths we know. Even in our multiplicity of differences and unique identities, we are all made of carbon, blood and stars.

Contemporary healers have an essential part to play in changing the world. I suspect you heal in your own particular way. I know you listen to the stories underneath the stories and ask the questions that discover. Your friends, coworkers and family seek a special kind of support from you, a medicine that you bring to the people whose lives you touch, even if you are not any kind of formal health care practitioner.

Julia Cameron, author of *The Artist's Way,* names this quality, "spiritual electricity". She says that we work with the divine when we cultivate our creativity and express it.[1] I call it your soul fire, the way that we plug our hands and hearts into the flow of the universe, whether we are fixing cars, bandaging wounds, studying the disappearance of frogs or playing the piano. When you are in the zone. When you feel something move through you. Whatever you call it, your medicine is the way you make things a little better than they were before you showed up. When you do that thing that you do, it heals us all.

You are exactly the kind of global revolutionary healer we have been waiting for. We must change our definition of healing to include all acts that seek to:

- Transform our world
- Release a commonly held vision of apocalyptic greed
- Repair the damage of desperate epidemic depression/anxiety/rage
- Diversify cooperation between cultures and all beings.

There is something that happens in the treatment room, the office, the classroom, the hospital that has a lasting effect. We see profound awakenings all the time at gatherings, conferences, music festivals, camping trips, workshops. It can happen anywhere.

We have scientists in our global revolutionary healer corner who pursue research that "acknowledges nutrition, emotion, and sustainable environments and recognizes that prayer, meditation, altruism, optimism, and forgiveness have a role in healing."[2] This is a giant shift in our cultural consciousness and one whose time has come.

Claire Hoertz Bardaracco, in her book, *Prescribing Faith,* says, "The National Institute of Health estimates that the number of visits to complementary medical care providers currently exceeds the number of visits to primary care physicians, a trend that has strengthened since NIH's first survey in 1990. Sixty-two percent of the 31,000 Americans surveyed in 2002 reported having used prayer as a Complementary and Alternative Medicine (CAM) therapy within the past year; prayer was among twenty other alternative practices listed as options, including meditation, yoga, reiki, tai chi, diet, vitamins, chiropractic, massage, biofeedback, energy healing, folk medicine, guided imagery, herbs and homeopathic treatment, hypnosis, progressive relaxation, qi gong, and deep breathing." Bringing a sacred context back into healing has aroused a great deal of interest in the contemporary urbanized world.[3]

The Old English *hāl* is the verbal root of the word heal, which actually means "to make whole." "Heal carries the meaning of restoration from an undesirable condition and at an elemental level pertains to saving, purifying, cleansing, and repairing to bring about restoration from...suffering or unwholesomeness."[5] We regularly refer to healing in reference to human physicality and psychology but the crucial meaning of the word covers the full revitalization of wholeness—to a holism of all beings in interdependence.

In Greek mythology, Chiron is a centaur, half horse and half human. In battle, he becomes wounded by a magical poison arrow and the wound will not heal no matter what treatment is given. Even with this significant setback, Chiron teaches the young healers and leaders, well known as the wounded healer. The story of Chiron reminds us that we cannot wait until we are perfect, even our wounds have power. People want healers who have done their own healing work, who understand what it is to be in that vulnerable position of needing care. Our own wounded healer stories are the best way to connect to the giant story of the earth and our evolving species.

I want to introduce you to nine key cross cultural healing practices. These nine sacred concepts are energetic truths that show up all over the globe, not borrowed from any particular culture without permission. They show up in our collective consciousness as humans. When we practice them, we overcome distraction, fear and disconnection in order to talk about spirit and medicine boldly.

I dare you to introduce one of them or all of them into your small corner of the modern world. Your contribution matters, more than you will ever know. Never assume there are enough of us already. If you are ready to claim your place as a global revolutionary healer, we need you. Please come and do that thing you do! I dare you to take a step towards the evolution of your inner healer and your unique medicine. It's time to dream the beginning of the world instead of the end.

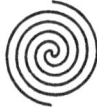

A Tale of a Spiritual Seeker

As a child, I experienced the earth around me as alive. In the green hills of Kentucky, I saw trees breathing and living spirits in the plants around me.

I lived in a lot of different houses growing up. One ritual I had to get to know a new neighborhood was to walk through and visit the trees that I really liked, even if they were in someone else's yard. The concept of my tree friends living in "someone else's yard" was strange to me. How could the trees belong to anyone but themselves? I spoke to them, sometimes drawing or naming them or writing stories about them. If I felt sad or disappointed, spending time outside always helped me feel better. Adults in my life commented on what a great imagination I had. As I grew older, I convinced myself that this had been a dream, talking plants were a fantasy or a metaphor.

In my early grades, I loved faery tales, poetry and mythology from all over the world. I also enjoyed the living sciences, especially biology, anatomy, geology, and psychology. Bringing creativity together with more formalized knowledge enticed me, as if they were two halves that desperately sought each other. I was excited by the spirit of scientific inquiry and solving the problems of the universe through experiments and observation. I also loved to tell stories and lugged stacks of books wherever I went. I was encouraged by my parents and teachers to write my own chronicles and anything else I could pour into the holy vessel of the blank page. I filled journal after journal.

My social studies teacher discussed peoples from other places who used creation myths to depict the beginning of the world or used story to explain what we now recognize to be scientific phenomenon. I got in trouble one day for asking if the stories of Adam and Eve in the Bible were a kind of creation myth. The teacher at my Catholic school was flustered. He assured me that it was not the same thing at all; these were true stories, not myths.[1]

I attended a different school each year for middle school. Puberty was brutal. I was shy, awkward in my body, and interested in academics. I felt mystified by the social systems that my classmates seemed to be constructing around who sat with whom at the lunch table.

I found solace in theatre training and fed my rich inner creative world. In performances we put together every few months, I told stories in a different way, using expressive art, movement, and voice to reveal different levels of reality. I was able to combat my shyness by pretending to be another character, if only for a short time.

My father moved out of our house. Divorce was cruel to my family, even when people were trying to do their best, I saw them at their worst. I was heartbroken to move again and leave my theatre troupe behind.

I did not have the energy or the interest to pursue theatre arts anymore. I began my struggle with depression. It became worse around romantic breakups or friendship upsets or anxiety about my perceived future but it was my constant companion.

In high school, my teachers showed us films about suicide with lots of reasons why we shouldn't want to die. There were vague American dream-esque possibilities of college, marriage, some kind of job, and kids, strong convincing presentations about why we should want to keep living.[2] Everything I valued was completely different from what I feared were my only options for the future. There was no room for mistakes. Everything depended on my perfection.

Why did I feel depressed when so many people on the planet had it much worse than I did? How dare I feel so miserable when I had enough to eat, clothes to wear, loyal friends, and a warm place to sleep at night? I tried to feel grateful for what was not happening to me and ignore what was feeling so difficult. My mother was working two jobs, my younger brother and I were each alone in our grief process.

I stayed away from home as much as possible. I scribbled my friends' names in my white diary locked and hidden underneath my mattress. I would be okay as long as other people liked me, I wouldn't disappear. I was never sure if my friends were really my friends, if anyone could really love me if they truly saw who I was. Depression was like carrying a backpack full of giant rocks around on your back. You could complete tasks with the pack on, but everything was much more challenging.

I quietly choked on my own fears and losses and it felt impossible to keep living that way. Who could I tell? Wouldn't they just run away if they knew me? The world did not welcome me. I had no place. Everyone seemed to be playing a game that I didn't understand.

Then, I met alcohol. Drinking after school, at parties anywhere I could was the mainstay of my social life. When I drank, I laughed with my friends. I forgot I was shy. Whenever I felt a tight, panicked feeling in my chest, I smoked a cigarette. Everything would relax; I could keep going.

I tried to get help. I told one school counselor that I was stressed out. She asked me to remember a time that I had been really happy. I told her about being a child and believing that the plants were alive and could talk. I told her about working in a theatre group to create performances. She asked me if I could cultivate that feeling in my life today. Was there a time I currently felt alive when I wasn't using substances? I couldn't think of anything. And it only got worse. It would be years before I dealt with my depression and addictive patterns. I would later learn to call this a dark night of the soul, and honor it as an initiatory opening to a healing path that I would walk for the rest of my life.

On a particularly bad night during my junior year in high school, I gave up and tried to take my own life. My suicide attempt was messy and desperate. If depression was my cage, trying to end my life was a prison break. It was not romantic. I did not succeed.

I ended up in the adolescent ward in the psychiatric hospital. Three weeks transpired like three years. I was hospitalized with twenty other teenagers who had recently attempted suicide.

We were fifteen, sixteen, fourteen, seventeen and hopeless. Our broken down brains betrayed us all the time, no longer producing what we needed for happiness.

There was the gracious girl with the paralyzed arm. she accidentally shot herself in the shoulder instead of the head.

The quiet boy who took a gun to school and held up the chemistry class that he was failing. He ordered a pizza and didn't shoot anyone.

The gorgeous girl who finally confronted her sexually abusive stepfather. her drunk mother beat her up and kicked her out so she walked in front of a car.

The thin boy whose father pushed him so hard to be athletic. he tried to hang himself when he didn't make the basketball team.

In the hospital, I didn't fake anything. There was nothing we could not say to each other. our strange and eclectic tribe formed from combined adolescent pain. We were teen super heroes from the halls of angst. In group therapy, we cared if someone's parent visit was horrible or if someone had a violent episode and went to the padded room or if someone found out their boyfriend cheated on them while they were locked up in the psych ward.

I met three other young women just like me and we became close so fast because we needed it so much. The hospital staff called us the "Four Musketeers" because we did everything together. It was so different to play the game of life with people on your team! I could live trembling, white knuckled and terrified, but I no longer had to do it alone.

One of the nurses' aides on our ward hung out with me in the sparse hospital library. A few times and we talked about survival and hope. He told me, "Girl, living is hard. It takes a lot of courage. I want you to get out of here and do great things with your life. I dare you to stay alive."

He made me want to learn to speak hope. Something inside me was stuck and I wanted to move it. I read every book I could find about people who survived. It didn't matter if it was about the Holocaust or The Color Purple. I had a lot of support from family and friends and I realized it wasn't true that I wanted to die. I wanted to come all the way back to life.

As a condition of my release from the hospital, I finally tried one of the SSRI antidepressant medications. I experienced a reprieve while on the medication; it was easier to exercise which lifted my depression and easier to feel hopeful. I was grateful for the motivation, but disappointed with the healing. The medication had terrible side effects. I hated the dull brain, dry mouth and dizziness that hit me at unexpected times so I stopped taking it. I wanted something more but I didn't know where to look. I promised myself and the people that I loved that I would keep living, but I wanted to do even more than that.

My resolve was tested over the next year and a half, when three of my friends from the hospital completed suicide, one after another.

Life outside the hospital was too hard. Not enough had changed for them. I wished I could have been more fluent in the language of hope to know how to save them. Why would they all leave me to face the world alone?

One night around this time, I had a dream where I sat in a sunny meadow with my best friends. We were surrounded by butterflies feasting on wildflowers and the butterflies came to rest on my hand, kissing my fingers. The scene switched and I stood in front of an empty YMCA swimming pool. An unseen person advised me to hold a piece of salami over the pool and sing my true name. When I did, a pair of rainbow colored, iridescent dolphins leapt out of the pool, gracefully taking turns eating the salami out of my hand until it was gone. And I sang the whole time.

I have always remembered that dream. Something inside me knew that I needed to believe in something beyond the ordinary to get through that difficult time.

The practice I carry from those years is one of allowing imperfect and awkward love from other people to enter my life, allowing all the beauty in. I practice asking for help, all the time, even when I don't think I need it. I am still fascinated with stories of survivors of all things, refugees, endangered species that reemerge, the ways that a burned and scorched forest yields seedlings. The world is so arbitrary that whether we live or die in any moment is uncertain. I cannot say what makes other people go on, but for me, it is the wonder, the magic that rips me open even when I think I am so crusted over, it could never happen again.

∞

SPECIAL LOVE NOTE FOR YOU tucked in here: When you struggle with who you are, how much you hurt and what your life means, please tell someone. We all deserve to break down the walls around the admission that we need help. Because when you leave this world, there is a terrible absence. I grieve the emptiness of the holes already left by those I have loved in my own clumsy, sporadic ways. I vow to keep inventing ways that we can reach for each other when we are falling, ways that we remember our true names and our places in this world, ways that we can sing ourselves and each other back to life, over and over. This is a revolution of the spirit.

∞

I went on to college to study pre-psychiatry. I searched for my own answers and attempted to bring the mysteries of the mind together with the needs of the body. I worked in a psychiatric hospital in Lexington, Kentucky, helping patients make art projects in the occupational therapy room. Randy always danced even when there was no music; Bill, an ex-NASA employee, said the government was evil and often did not get out of bed. Sheila wished she could stop hearing the voices and see her son graduate from eighth grade. I witnessed medication reduce symptoms for folks who were experiencing breaks with reality, but that wasn't enough to heal them. Something else was needed, and that didn't seem to live inside a pill.

One friendly dark-haired psychiatrist loved to stop by and admire the pottery we were making. She told me that often, medication was prescribed as the only solution to mental health challenges, especially with the rising levels of control that insurance companies had. They could dictate the entire treatment plans for individuals seeking mental health care, even if the doctor wanted something else.[3] I decided that I did not want to become a psychiatrist.

Toward the end of college, I cut down on drinking as my only means of entertainment. I hiked whenever I could. The Red River Gorge, one of the jewels of Kentucky, was about an hour's drive from my apartment. I explored its trails, creeks, and natural arches every weekend. I felt closer to health and remembered some of the joy I felt as a child, when I could talk to trees.

I started to meditate, experimenting with Buddhism, Taoism, and earth-based spirituality. I sought a source of spirituality that was not rigid or intolerant and that did not denigrate other faiths. I was interested in a God that was universal and personal, and broader than the white guy with a long white beard up in the sky. I questioned the gender of God. Why couldn't there be a female version of divinity or a deity of another race that could relate to me personally? I also wanted a spirituality that supported the gorgeous planet with whom I was falling in love again.

I moved to New Mexico to attend graduate school. I lived near mountains that glowed watermelon pink every day at sunset. I was 21 and desperate to know what I wanted to be when I grew up if not a doctor of psychiatry. I decided to get my Ph.D. as a clinical psychologist. The tuition would be greatly reduced if I were a New

Mexico resident. I took a job as a social worker in Albuquerque to live in town for a year and earn my in- state residency.

I sank into a world of endless blue skies, dry air, and green chile and cholla cacti. I fell asleep at night listening to coyote song. In my social work job, I developed specialized foster care programs for children and adults who had developmental disabilities. It was a good life.

New Mexico was a rich blend of culture. White people were definitely in the minority which broke up some of the homogeny of big-box store consumer culture that settled into many other places in the United States. There were many modalities of healing available to anyone who sought them and schools for every kind of healing work that you could imagine. People practiced traditional medicines freely, merging remedies from their grandmothers with modern innovations.

I learned a lot about Hispanic/Latino and Native American living traditions of healing and spirituality. I met people whose family members were *curanderas*, native New Mexican healers. My friends told me *curanderas* "talked" to plants and worked within a different kind of healing paradigm than what was offered in the hospitals. The healer in me was fascinated. What did they do that was so different than modern doctors?

I had neither Latina nor Native American heritage. My own ancestry being a mix of Western and Eastern Europe, I did not feel that I truly had access to learning these medicines. There were no schools and though folks were very willing to talk to me, the medicine was traditionally passed through family lineage.

One afternoon, my friend invited me to meet her aunt, a *curandera* in northern New Mexico. We ate sopapillas and watched the birds in her backyard. She nodded at me.

"It makes sense that you want to learn to heal in this older way. A long time ago, Europeans used to heal people in different ways too. It is sad for all of us that they do not anymore."

I was fascinated. I had not thought about what traditional medicine had looked like in Europe. Who were the folk healers of ancient Europe? Where were their unbroken traditions of herbal lore, of interpreting dreams, of easing grief, of midwifery practices? When had the systems that we now know as Western medicine come into being? What had happened to indigenous healing knowledge from Europe?

In History classes, I had read about the witch trials in Europe that went on for hundreds of years. They consumed women, children, and men, throwing the entire continent into fear of irrational accusations. I had seen it as a tragedy. I had never thought about it as a systematic assault on traditional healers.

Because I was trained as a scientist, I did what any scientist would do in my situation—research. In my research, I realized that to call a healer a *witch* and put her on trial was a clever way to discredit indigenous European spirituality. An accusation of witchcraft and the subsequent murders also created a centralized medical structure that excluded women and the former traditional health care.

No healers of that time would have used *witch* to self-describe, even if they were actually practicing indigenous European religions and celebrating festivals that honored the agricultural cycle. People may have called themselves "cunning folk" or "healers." The word *witch* was an insult, a word to strike fear into people's hearts and scare them away from the practice of medicine or the possibility of speaking their minds.

The land-based spirituality practiced in most parts of Europe may certainly have informed these healing practices. There was necessarily a connection to land and to the body as sacred. Those who sought to disavow these healers associated this land-based spirituality with devil worship and danger.

The association of devil worship with the practice of native European religion was erroneous, a leftover from the genocide that the governments of the Middle Ages ordered and the witch hunters enacted. The accusations of devil worship went on to be used to justify the African slave trade in the US as well as hundreds of years of the denigration of indigenous healing traditions on almost every continent. It was high time that modern culture separated these negative connotations from the word *witch* and acknowledged what happened to these native healing traditions.

It was not necessary or respectful for me to attempt to gain access to Native American or Latina folk healing unless someone freely gave it to me. I could research my own blood connection to land-based healing traditions. How did people of my ancestry practice holistic medicine? There was a world of Old European spiritual healing traditions that people were attempting to reconstruct from what was left after the Burning Times or recreate based on what had survived in other places. There was absolutely nothing evil about these practices. In understanding this, the world cracked open for me.

I studied what I could find of native European healing traditions including herbal lore, dream work, mythology, alchemy, divination, energy work, trance, ritual, mysticism, music, soul retrieval, and other healing practices. I also found the beauty and mysticism of my religion of origin, Catholicism. The sacred and devotional practices of most religions were not the same as the beliefs that humans used to beat each other over the head or kill each other in holy wars. There were energetic truths in all these traditions whose purpose was to awaken a sense of connection, wonder, and joy. All rivers flowed back to the same sea.

My favorite name for what I believe and practice is nature-centered spirituality. The divine is all around us; there is wonder embedded in the natural cycles, the seasons, the life and death of all beings. The Earth is alive and we are interdependent with our planet. I am inspired by spiritual traditions from all over the world, particularly the multiplicity of the paths which hold sacred the beliefs that joy and healing, justice and transformation are vital parts of human life.

In the first few months of my job as a social worker in Albuquerque, I became ill with a terrible chest cold that morphed into bronchitis, or possibly pneumonia. I did not have health insurance. It would be three months before my new benefits began. I treated myself with herbs and over-the-counter cough syrup for a few weeks but nothing seemed to help. The cough got worse, the mucous became thick and dark. The visit to the doctor who might prescribe antibiotics was more than I could afford. I coughed all night. I was scared.

My neighbor across the street attended acupuncture school and urged me to make an appointment at the student clinic at Southwest Acupuncture College. I wanted anything that would help. The student intern spoke with me for a few minutes and then ran to fetch her supervisor, a Chinese woman, small in stature with a stern voice. "You have an evil qi invasion," she proclaimed. She proceeded to treat me with acupuncture needles and glass cups that she warmed with fire and placed on my back to pull out the evil qi. She bled the corners of my fingernails with lancets to release the heat inside me. I was exhausted after the treatment and slept for hours.

I woke up the next morning to a faint cough with clear mucous. I could breathe! In two days, I felt normal. I read everything I could about this miraculous medicine. A few months later, I registered for a graduate program to become a Doctor of Oriental Medicine.

The Chinese character for medicine (yao) has its basis in the Chinese character for music. Medicine, like music, is meant to bring the body back into harmony, restore its unique sound.[4] In medical school, our teachers told us that the body is seen as a series of pathways or meridians that are roads for a substance called *qi* (pronounced "chee"). Qi cannot be measured or quantified. It is the life force and also the way that cells communicate with each other. It is accessed easily at certain points on the meridians. These are the places where acupuncturists insert hair-like needles. Health is based on the flowing movement of qi. When the qi is stuck or deficient, bodies experience pain or disease. The acupuncturist helps the patient by moving the stagnant qi at the sites where the needles are placed, relieving pain, and reminding the body of a flowing pattern of health.

At the foundation of Chinese Medicine theory, there are five elements that correspond to body systems. Each element has correspondences to physical, emotional, and spiritual qualities. *(see figure 1)*

Along with the movement of qi, another goal of Chinese medicine is to determine which element is in play or out of balance in the person's pattern or chief complaint. Acupuncture points are related to the elements, so if the person's Earth element is low, we might treat the digestive system, choosing points on the Spleen and Stomach meridians to bring ease to the body (see diagram). For a patient with depression, we could focus on the Wood element and remove the barriers to a new vision of life.

In school, I learned to recognize patterns and prescribed acupuncture points related to various disorders. Each needle was uniquely applied. If two patients came into the clinic with digestive difficulties, an acupuncturist might treat them in two different ways based on their other symptoms and the quality of their pulses.

I kept finding inklings of the spiritual truths that I suspected had been obscured from the medicine I was now learning. One teacher asked our class to increase the sensitivity in our fingers so that we could "feel" the qi at the acupuncture points from the outside. She suggested that we take a hair from our heads and put it in a phone book or another large book with very thin pages. We were then to turn the pages slowly over the hair and see how many pages we could turn and still feel the hair beneath them. All of us wanted to sense the qi coursing beneath the skin, a mystical life

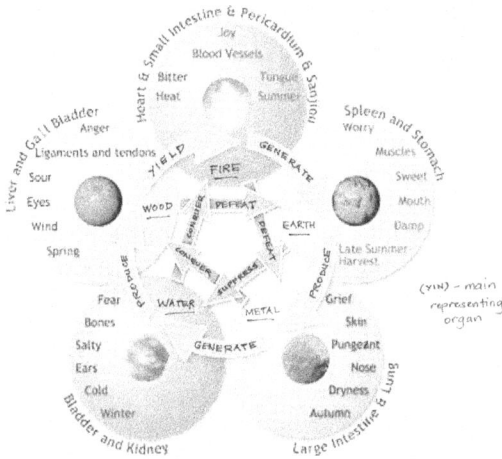

FIG. 1

force that we were learning to guide. We heard stories of masters who could move qi with their fingers alone and breathing techniques that could increase longevity and happiness.

In Chinese medicine, we checked for more than just the rates of the pulses. We felt the quality of the pulse and used an ancient system of reading the health of all the body systems through the pulse. It was never formulaic or cut-and-dried. The pulses always seemed as complex as the human being in front of me. I started some meditative practices before I approached my patients, to ask quietly to hear the story of the pulse, as if the pulse was the headline giving me the news of the current events of the person I was treating.

Qi and blood flow together through the body. The language of qi can be found in the chemical impulses shared during inflammation responses to an injury. When we are irritated or grieving, it is qi that makes up the emotions. The expression of the emotion moves the qi in our bodies.

Yet, no one can say definitively what qi is or measure it with a lab test. There are now scientific studies and research to prove that biochemical markers change in people's bodies when needles are inserted. There is a lot of conjecture about why acupuncture works but its mechanisms remain mysterious. For some, that is a challenge to do more research and discover the cause and effect relationships in a way that cannot be discounted by naysayers of acupuncture. For me, it feels unlikely that there will ever be a measurement of qi that speaks to its true nature. It would always be more poetry than accounting. That never bothered me about the medicine. I received early training in theater and creative writing as well as in scientific research. I knew art when I saw it. However, it became clear in my schooling that the history of the medicine was conflicted about the science versus the art of it.

Early Chinese medicine saw humans as fundamentally part of the earth, not separate from it. Prevention of disease was vital. An emphasis on moderation in diet and healthful lifestyle habits helped people live long lives. "The good doctor pays constant attention to keeping people well so that there will be no sickness" said Huai Nan-tzu, an ancient Chinese doctor and philosopher.[6] Exercise, deep breathing, dietary recommendations, and sleep were often the first course of action to treat people in ancient China.

Chinese medicine was influenced at its roots by Taoism, alchemy, Siberian shamanism, Confucianism, Buddhism and many other forms of spirituality. The Maoist revolution in China in the 1940–1970s, took the story of this medicine in another direction. Many sources describe the purposeful driving underground of the native spirituality inherent in the medicine that was practiced until that time, dismissing it as folklore. There was a sacred context in this "Classical" Chinese Medicine that had been separated from the Traditional Chinese Medicine that I was now learning. Many of these lost teachings were similar to what had been buried in the European healing traditions by a similar attack on healers.

The intentions behind the exile of the practitioners of Chinese medicine seemed to be to help people receive legitimate medicine and to protect them from suspected charlatans. In the 1940s, Mao Zedong became disdainful of the theories of yin and yang and suspicious of the five elements. He decreed that people were practicing magic, shamanism, and worse or that they were complete dilettantes, taking advantage of people who were ill. Even though Mao himself was taking herbal formulas to prevent respiratory infections, he made the practice of Chinese medicine illegal in 1942.[7]

Practitioners were forced to go into hiding. Their books and supplies, if found, were burned or destroyed by the communist Red Guard. In some situations, healers were killed or sentenced to indoctrination camps to change their ways of thinking.[8] There was no blending of best practices from the former practitioners with the newly emerging variety of medicine that the Maoists favored.

Every effort was made to eradicate the practices of the knowledge and the wisdom that had gone before.

This reliance on science was the impetus for an influx of Western style medicine coming to China in the late '60s and early '70s. This medicine was believed to be successful and efficient. A blended style of Western medicine and what became known as "Traditional Chinese Medicine" was born. This TCM was effective, using rigorous theory and the scientific method and recipe prescription for acupuncture points. However, there was an absence of the art and spirituality immanent in the kind of medicine that was practiced pre-Mao.

In the long shadow of attacks on healing like the Cultural Revolution or the Burning Times, the imprint of our culture's prevailing values says that to offer a mixture of spirituality and health in an urbanized culture is either inane or dangerous. Healing must only be a matter of cause and effect or a discussion of the appearance of symptoms and their elimination. Anything else is clearly a manifestation of devil worship, circus entertainment, or attempted snake oil sales. This may still be the party line, but many healers and patients alike are shouting that this is a small-minded, obsolete reduction of the actual truth about our personal and collective health.

Acupuncturists, chiropractors, osteopaths, massage therapists, naturopaths, midwives, and other kinds of healers have had to fight to practice their medicine legally, or to be able to participate in the insurance systems. There is still a great tension perceived between allopathic and complementary medicines in Western culture, including Chinese medicine. Many acupuncturists have worked to make acupuncture available without doctor referrals, covered by insurance plans, and available in low-cost clinics. Sometimes acupuncturists participate in the fear that talking about anything esoteric might drive people away. So we continue the work of the Maoists and pretend that the medicine we practice is not spiritual in nature or that we have evolved beyond that kind of medicine in pursuit of more measurable outcomes.

Yet, the billions spent out of pocket on health care not covered by insurance companies caused a reevaluation of what kinds of treatments are covered and available. Medical schools now offer courses that investigate spirituality's relationship to health care. Patients see more options than simply turning themselves over to the hands of a physician who endeavors to cure them with more and more medications and surgeries, if this approach does not yield results.

A folk saying from Chinese medicine's history is "The good physician first cures the disease of the nation, then human ailments."[9] The transformation of this culture will take more than laser surgeries and stronger antibiotics. At my graduation from Chinese medical school, our professional oath had a line that read: "I will live and practice medicine for people rather than for things. Empathy for my patients will never be subservient to skill and knowledge." It further read: "I will motivate and assist others to strengthen their health, reduce risk of disease, and preserve the health of the planet for ourselves, our families, and future generations."[10] There is a challenge here for global revolutionary healers, should we choose to accept it. The experiment would be to trust that it is time to bring our kind of medicine to the public.

In a World Healing Exchange trip to Nepal with Acupuncturists Without Borders in 2013, our teams treated over 500 people in community clinics that we set up throughout Kathmandu and the northern region of Mustang. We rode horses from village to village like circus performers. There were mountains that could steal your breath, the color of sand, silver, blood, cinnamon and rust. We rode past fields of green tsampa barley that pretended to be oceans when the wind gusted through the Kali Ghandaki River valley. We used the NADA protocol, five acupuncture points found in the ears that reset the nervous system, healing trauma and post-traumatic stress.

In Nepal, I was told that Namaste meant "the god in me greets the god in you." We were encouraged to ardently greet the divine in everyone we met. And sure enough, there was brightness, a clear window into something living there.

I have been looking for the gods in other people since I have returned. I look for that fire in their eyes, in their movement, in the body of energy that travels before them like weather. The gods here in the U.S. may be sleeping or fetal or distracted by iPhones. I can't demand their company, but I will offer Namaste as a dare, a gambit, something risky. I love to watch humans glow with that divine kindling that fills each of us. That is the grace that can save our creative spirit and lead us away from the greedy, empty edge of the land of zombies.

We need all the tools we can possibly acquire to help each other recover from trauma, fully heal from injury, and remember what is beautiful about our lives. Here we go.

CHAPTER ONE

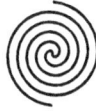

Medicine with Soul and Spirit

Why
Just ask the donkey in me
To speak to the donkey in you,
When I have so many other beautiful animals
And brilliant colored birds inside...
Let's hold hands and get drunk near the sun
And sing sweet songs to God
Until He joins us with a few notes
From his own sublime lute and drum.

— HAFIZ

In my early twenties, I end a relationship and lose a friendship. I suddenly develop frequent migraine headaches that cause intense pain and nausea. It's not QUITE the same as the old weight of depression; I know that I will get through it. This is not the worst thing in the world. I will feel better eventually. Still, everything in my life feels gray and grief throbs. After several weeks of moping around the house, I go to hear Bernie Worrell, the keyboard player for Parliament and the Talking

Heads in concert. His keyboard music is a blend of jazz, funk, and a kind of lightness that I had forgotten. In dancing, I release something heavy and raw. In dancing, I take flight and feel the laughter rise through my pores. In the music, something heals me. I find a crazy joy within my body and remember why life matters.

My acupuncture patient goes to her doctor to inquire about treatment for debilitating migraines that are compromising her ability to work and enjoy her family. The doctor prescribes medication that relieves the pain but makes her feel sick, spacey, and intoxicated. She returns to his office after a few weeks to talk about the side effects of the medication. She asks about lifestyle changes, other options for treatment, dietary recommendations, stress relief techniques but is given no information or referrals. She is told that taking the medication is the only thing that she can do to treat her headaches.

Sacred Exploration

In the world in which we live, it is considered normal to work as much as possible, get little exercise because we are too tired and too busy, and eat food that is processed and full of additives. We are often more curious about the people we watch on television than what is happening in our neighborhoods. My professional development and acupuncture clients constantly describe a lack of energy. Sometimes I feel that myself.

There is research and rhetoric about the effects of stress on bodies and emotions, but very little in the way of treatment or long-term ways to reduce stress. We are living in an epidemic of depression, anxiety, and post-traumatic stress syndrome. Our bodies dump adrenaline, norepinephrine, and cortisol into our systems in traffic jams, meetings, and sometimes, while we read email messages. We connect to each other through phone calls and the internet. We are more isolated than humans have ever been.

It is hard to say when the trend of disembodiment and disassociation in our culture began. Much has been written on the separation between body and spirit and the transcendental beliefs that locate God out there in heaven and name the earth a silent inanimate rock. The Protestant work-ethic is another contributor to this disassociation, the idea that humans are lowly worms, worthless unless we provide, work, or produce. Many of us are taught in modern culture that we must work hard for our money and that our wealth is measured by what we own or where we can afford to go.

As an urban civilization, we focus on crafting and maintaining our image. Consumer culture and the media take turns dangling shiny carrots in front of us. We are motivated to buy conspicuous designer clothing, shiny, fast, trendy vehicles, or any number of items in order to make ourselves more beautiful or display our wealth. Ads convince us that our bodies are too fat/thin, too tall/short, too pale/dark and that there are numerous ways to spend our money to remedy these failings. Advertising assures us that we can escape our ailments, our insecurities, and our ennui with more, new and better stuff. A culture of people who were pretty darn happy with themselves just the way they were would cause a major upset to this industry.

In my acupuncture practice, I often give patients the metaphor of the labor movement to describe our bodies. It is hard to admit to our having been sometimes cruel or unthinking supervisors to our own bodies. It can be difficult to imagine our body systems functioning as workers who often are not fed well, who are asked to labor long hours sometimes under terrible conditions, for little reward, and aren't allowed to sleep long enough. Our bodies can't always do what our minds want them to do. Then, we become upset that our expectations are not met. We continue to force our bodies to do things of which they are not capable. Often, we do not feed them well or give them the rest that might help get them back on track. Yet, when our bodies go on strike, we have very little recourse.

To provide the majority of medicine for many people in first world countries, a force of doctors has been created who specialize in prescribing medications and performing surgical procedures. This has been incredibly beneficial for many reasons.

Because of chemotherapy and antibiotics, people with access to medicines do not always die of cancer or septic infections. Numerous illnesses and conditions that used to threaten death or disfigurement have been all but conquered. Contracting HIV is not necessarily a death sentence anymore, at least for those who have access to the medicine that keeps AIDS from developing. If an organ inside the body stops functioning, modern medicine can transplant another one and save a life. If some part of the body is troubled, often, a surgery can remove it or manipulate the tissue to work better. Sometimes this kind of excision is helpful and necessary, but other times, there is another form of healing for which the body asks.

Modern medicine took the knowledge of health care out of the hands of indigenous healers and folk remedies that elders or grandparents could administer. It is at least partially true that the advent of the internet has given back some of that access to medical information to the general public. But a lot of traditional medicines are dying out or being dismissed as ineffective.

There are many ingredients that complete the picture of health care. What if the solution is not an either/or but a more radical inclusion of something else?

The word *spirit* is not new. We find its roots in the Latin word, *spiritus,* which also blooms into words such as inspiration, and the very embodied words, respiration and perspiration. There are psychological and religious connotations of spirit, images of gurus and mountain peaks, disembodied voices speaking from above. Many folks these days identify as spiritual rather than religious; one of the reasons for this may be to escape rigid definitions of what God is and is not.

I define spirit as an ineffable essence that lives in all things, the collective life force that inhabits what is animate. Our definitions of what is animate may vary, but if you see the life force in it, an argument can be made that it is alive in some sense. Does a mossy rock have life force? Does a shopping mall? A waterfall? A sculpture? A pigeon? A train station? In which of these do you find more spirit? Which of them connects you more with the holism of life?

The spirit is the source where our personal consciousness joins with a larger life force, whether this is some form of God or a collective human consciousness. We can call this our divinity or our numinous self, but I will refer to it as our spirit. In ancient Egyptian hieroglyphics and medieval art, artists painted a glowing nimbus around the head of the figure to symbolize the connection of each figure with the sacred.

Is it the numinous life force itself that is missing from our medicine and our daily routines? How did we get this way? How do we remove the blocks to this enlivening spirit? What can we do to come back to ourselves and unlock our human potential? What if body, mind, soul, and spirit were able to reintegrate in some fundamental way?

James Hillman (1926–2011), a brilliant depth psychologist and author, warned us against preferring an abstract version of spirit to the more tangible soul that he defined as the sum of daily experiences. Hillman's soul is much like Carl Jung's anima, or the "archetype of life." Hillman denigrated any spiritual experience that is too transcendent, that does not ground us in matter, in the tangibles of daily living. "It is not the trip and its stations…not the rate of ascent and the rung of the ladder, or the peak and its experiences, nor even the return—it is the person in the person prompting the whole endeavor."[1] It is impossible to simply transcend ourselves and escape our lives. Our lives are real; they happen in a place and they are based in activity and relationship.

For me, the soul is the more primal part of us, the way that humans are ancient animals as well as conscious thinkers. The soul is interwoven with the visions of the mind, the intelligence of the body, and the voice of the emotions. This is why we often talk about "heart and soul." The individual soul is an integral part of the spirit, and its inclusion completes any healthy spirituality. Our spirit is the divine part of us, our soul is the primal part of us, and both are intertwined in our human heart that holds our emotions and thoughts and our human body that encapsulates us and provides our home.

Perhaps there is not such a great a difference between spirit and soul if our goal is to move toward a more embodied spirituality. The separation seems strained at best and it is hard to tell where the dividing line might be if we are fully living in our body, mind and spirit as holistic beings. This feels significant when we begin to speak of the coming revolution of the spirit. If spirit and soul originate within each of us and their connection to the larger Spirit can be developed, then perhaps our internal landscapes can be trained to mirror the expressions of divine beauty that we find outside of us. Would this bring us closer to collective health?

James Hillman talked about the ways that we define the edges of our human experience. Where does what you consider "you" stop and what you consider "the world" begin? He believed that people who have very close relationships to the land on which they live may make the boundary of self much further away from their individual, physical body than folks who live in an urban setting.

The ways that we connect or disconnect from the life force or from the larger reality of our ecosystem may have a profound effect on our health in the long term. The ways that we do or do not identify ourselves with what is around us may also play into our well-being. It is very difficult to make changes in our environment if we do not consider it part of us. [2]

In my own search for the sacred, the more I opened to the possibility of something larger than myself, the more I began to have spiritual or at least connective experiences with many of the elements that our European ancestors believed to be divine, especially air, fire, water, and earth. In Chinese Medicine, these elements were also revered as essential parts of the human body, mind, spirit as well as being primal forces of nature.

Living in the New Mexico desert opened me to the power of water, the absolute love of it. Water fills any vessel we construct, the original shape-shifter. When there was serious drought, I learned to pray for the rain. I turned my parched face to the clouds and wished I knew the secret to open the door to the heavens. I understood why native people included water in their worship. Acknowledging my interdependence with water helped me to remember that my own life's pattern was not set in stone, perhaps it was even more "fluid" than I believed. Water asked me to live in a different way, to trust, to surrender to the flow of something that I could not control.

When I moved from Albuquerque to Portland, Oregon, my relationship with water changed significantly. Though I celebrated the fact that water came effortlessly from the sky in the temperate rain forests of the Pacific Northwest, it took some getting used to. I had ridiculous expectations of the rain, wanting it to feed my garden but never ruin a hike. I struggled with feeling sluggish, laden with the weight of the cloud ceiling. It became my instinct to duck my head while dashing through drizzle. I shuddered when the icy drops hit my skin and moved slightly faster to escape my adversary. I invested in a Gore-Tex raincoat so that I could go about my business, even on the dampest of mornings, and remain impervious.

After a year of resenting the rain, on an unseasonably warm October evening, I decided to strip off my Gore-Tex jacket and join the torrents. I tasted the rain, letting it sting my face and dampen me. I stood in the yard and then dried off and sat on the porch for an hour, listening to the recital. The rain commenced with a downpour and swelled to a deluge. From that crescendo, it softened to drizzly mist. I went to bed with lesser drips pinging against the gutter, resonant in the deep gray night.

After that, I adopted water as my medium, no longer ducking my head, but meeting it with unswerving resolve. I waved to my neighbors and inquired after their days even when it was raining. I whispered prayers of gratitude for the pregnancy of our garden and the health of the forests. The lessons of water for me were the same—trust, surrender, and give thanks.

Not everyone is looking for experiences of the sacred in their medicine. Not everyone wants to commune outside with the elements. I feel delight when someone comes in my office with back pain that has no deeper somatic meaning. I see many patients who come in with muscle sprains or injuries that heal easily and they are ready to reenter their lives just as they were. However, those people do not begrudge my other patients the opportunity to transform deeper injuries, to reconnect to themselves, and to bring more spirituality into their everyday experience.

The fact that anyone would begrudge another their choice of healing path is a major part of the problem that we face. Taking a spiritual history could help health care practitioners determine what the spiritual needs of their patients are and what kinds of support are necessary and welcome. "When terminal illness or serious surgeries are involved, doctors ought to learn their patients' perception....When religion conflicts with prescriptions, transfusions, or other interventions... it becomes even more important to understand spiritual histories." [3]

What do we as a culture fear about bringing the possibility of body, mind, and spirit back into our medicine? Why is spirituality in health care a political issue?

Religions that do not embrace a single God or exist outside the Judeo-Christian paradigms are still not considered legitimate spiritual traditions in many places. The threat of being burned at the stake has diminished in some places as religious freedom rises, but there is still a fear of being thought of as dangerous for many folks who choose to follow indigenous spiritual paths or receive care from a practitioner of traditional medicine. There still seems to be an overarching opinion that these traditions are less serious or are hokey, foolish, and ridiculous. What is the underlying fear here?

In this area, the eradication of indigenous European healers and midwives haunts us still. The systems of herbal lore that were lost were useful in preventative care as well as in natural childbirth, menstrual care, and pain management. The setback to midwifery as a practice continues to be a struggle for people in Western countries who have healthy pregnancies and want to give birth at home or at birthing centers. It is also quite challenging for those who are called to be midwives where the state laws only support hospital births and give preference to the frequently scheduled cesarean sections that may not be medically necessary.[4]

The identification of healing, midwifery, and indigenous spiritual practices of native Europeans with evil magic was a diabolically strategic move. Thousands of people, mostly women, were tortured or killed and their land dispersed among other landowners. It also gave missionaries an easy way to continue to spread their work abroad and cast suspicion on all indigenous religious and healing practices for years to come. The accusation of someone practicing witchcraft still carries a heavy legal penalty or a severe social stigma in many countries today.

It was vital in the Europe of the sixteenth and seventeenth centuries to systematically change the identity of the familiar women who lived and worked in the villages into something alien or demonic. The agenda of the leadership at that time was expansion into the West and there was an influx of financial and political difficulty at home. No wonder this period earned the nickname, the Age of Anxiety! There had to be a clearly identified enemy on which to focus. The use of the label, "witch" allowed the creation of a model for evil so that Europeans could compare themselves to this and be morally upright. This then allowed them to participate in the slave trade, murder local healers, and conquer indigenous peoples abroad while avoiding any kind of moral self-scrutiny. [5]

The Puritan colonists sailed to America with dreams of freedom from religious oppression. Yet, those who experience suffering often repeat it. The witch trials in Salem and other towns of the Northeast are well known. Anyone who practiced other religious beliefs than Puritanism in the early days of European settlers coming to America, were often ridiculed, accused of witchcraft, or had their businesses boycotted. Quakers and Native Americans were regularly targeted as well as anyone who practiced healing or spirituality of native Europe. It wasn't enough that the Puritans believed what they believed. Everyone else had to practice it too or perish.

We may not be as overt with our cultural prejudices around healing these days, but we also have a lot of work to do in acknowledging the aftershock effects of Puritanism in our current medical practices. Bringing spirituality back to healing would require modern healers to be vigilant about their own intolerance or judgment about others' beliefs and spiritual practices.

The archetype of healer is as old as the development of human society. The Bible describes Jesus as a great healer, a performer of miracles. The Navajo people believe that when people are divided from the healthy flow of life force, a healer must assist them in their return.[6] The Chinese Taoists developed an entire system of medicine to do just that. Every society has had their healers, their medicine people, their physicians, their nurses, wise women, caregivers, and shamans. Often, the cures that were provided were meant to work not only on a physical level but also addressed psychological, spiritual, political, and environmental damages.

A study by Schmidt suggests that healers can hold an intention and a presence that are imperative to the therapeutic process for the patient.[7] In this view, healers are not interchangeable; the chemistry and trust between the person being healed and the healer are valuable. Schmidt states that "the doctor needs to communicate to the patient a spiritual attitude of unconditional love, acceptance, and positive regard and this cannot occur when the healer has not yet developed that dimension of mindfulness. The role of humor and laughter has been documented in the mind-body literature as therapeutic, but when applied to the healing presence of doctors, the humor needs to be more subtle and to communicate the mystic's message that all will be well, even in the face of serious illness—that the doctor is not judging the patient in any way but accepting the sufferer as someone who once was well, just like the doctor is today...Acceptance of the patient's reality and the ability to separate the patient from the illness...are attributes of a physician's healing presence."[8]

A revolution of the spirit in medicine would make all kinds of religion, all spirituality welcome in our health care, with no preference for a single one and no pressure on people to choose to be spiritual at all if that is not their preference.

We have grounds to question our unflagging dependence on technical, precise, and systematic results as the only way that anyone could ever help a person to heal. We believe our current system of medical care is based in the Enlightenment (or Age of Reason) of European history when the scientific method came along to create a logical way to get reproducible results. While this way of studying data is useful and often quite practical, it is not a complete picture of healing. It is necessary to have trials to test medications and theories must be tested to see if results can be replicated. However, the scientific method can't always explain why some people get well and some die, even with the same type of treatment. We can't explain why some medicines work on some people and some don't. We discard any healing results that cannot be readily explained, mumbling about the power of placebo and discarding symptoms that don't respond to medication or surgery as "psychosomatic." This is incredibly shortsighted. There are far more ways to know things than proving them through the scientific method. Many of those ways could be valuable to our practices and our patients.

We must keep asking how our current way of practicing medicine in the dominant Western world is working. What is the best care that we can give to people?

Even beyond statistics, sample studies, and anecdotes, many people in the Western world would agree that there is something absent from their medical care. Happiness and healing still feel far away for many people in urbanized culture. There is something missing.

Margaret Wills asserts, "The recognition that spirituality is a valid component of healthcare seems to be today's breaking news."[9] The post-Enlightenment consensus seemed to be that science had the solutions to health concerns and that spirituality had no place in the treatment room. This is being challenged in studies that the NIH has funded since the 1990s on the connections between mind and body, faith and healing. The Alcoholics Anonymous movement has long since claimed a relationship to a higher power is a key ingredient in transforming addictive patterns. In 2003, studies found that one third of Americans over eighteen years of age have sought answers to health challenges and illness from "various non-mainstream sources including spiritual practices.[10] However, many practitioners still suspect that Complementary and Alternative Medicine (CAM) is currently the only place where spirituality can be addressed or discussed without fear of losing legitimacy in the eyes of the public.

Many of the practices that have been adopted by people in the Western world to combat stress and illness have originated in the spiritual traditions of other countries. Yoga, tai qi, martial arts, meditation, more progressive and holistic forms of counseling all come to us from spiritual traditions that value mystery and touch the source of something original. Calling it a connection to God or other deities may be less important than the translation of the mystery to the human experience.

In March of 2000, the White House established a commission to investigate the benefits of a more holistic approach to health care, potentially including Complementary and Alternative Medicine as legitimate sources for healing. Their report in 2002 clearly states that "Health involves all aspects of life-mind, body and spirit and environment—and high-quality health care must support care of the whole person."[11]

There seems to be no question in the research that spirituality can be an important contributor to health and recovery from illness. Studies from the early 2000s on varied spiritual practices from Catholicism, Islam, Hinduism, and Christianity show that spirituality factors into healing, whether the research took place through self-reporting, focus groups, or rating efficacy on a scale.[12] The definition of spirituality, not connected to any single religion, also seems to be important. In Piedmont's Spiritual Transcendence Scale, some commonalities between diverse faiths were found. A definition of spirituality is applied to healing as an active, hopeful, and connective process.[13] Weaker identification with spirituality, regardless of faith, seems to leave people closer to a passive, hopeless, separate experience on a spectrum of healing outcomes.

In a spiritual healing process, people are actively engaged in seeking their own wellness. "People assume personal responsibility for themselves and their health."[14] Doctors are not necessarily seen as the bringers of cures and the patient is not a passive recipient of a diagnosis or illness. The research continues to indicate that people who have more spiritual lives seem to focus on the healing process and "healing does not mean going back to the way things were before and is not the same as curing."[15] Healing in a spiritual context is not a one-time isolated phenomenon, but an ongoing active and unfolding process that leaves us hopeful that we can survive and thrive and find joy again.

Whether healer or patient, spirit is what we are seeking in our healing processes. It is the experience of magic, mystery, the unknown joy that we want. Our lack of happiness and holistic health is due to the spiritual anorexia that is a long-term side effect of a Puritan heritage. We live with an intolerant social construct that we have not formally abandoned.

We can abandon it now.

CHAPTER TWO

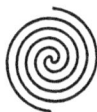

Embodiment: The Voice of the Body

The Church says: The body is a sin.
Science says: The body is a machine.
Advertising says: The body is a business.
The body says: I am a fiesta.

— EDUARDO GALEANO

◇◇◇

I walk home from work at night in quiet mist. The city streets are almost empty. I sense the man behind me, following too close. My heart strikes syncopated rhythms. My vision crystallizes my muscles prime to run. My thoughts assure me that I probably have nothing to fear. I cross the street anyway. The man does not follow me.

◇◇◇

My patient goes into the breast cancer clinic to speak to her oncologist about her reaction to chemotherapy. She is frustrated by many of the symptoms she is experiencing since taking the chemo. The port for the chemotherapy inserted near her clavicle is red and inflamed, possibly infected. Her energy is low and she is depressed. The nurse listens and does not have much to offer in the way of advice. My client repeats her words to me later, "We do a good job of getting rid of the cancer but don't do as well taking care of the whole person."

Sacred Exploration:

The ability to remain present within our bodies, grounded in time and space, sounds as if it would be effortless. And yet, much of our early social training teaches us to ignore information from our senses in order to learn polite behaviors. Bodies instantly decide if a situation is safe or dangerous, whether we are attracted or repulsed by a person. Our bodies are the last remnants of our wild nature. Our sympathetic nervous system responds automatically to stress without having to plan a reaction. In a healthy body, the parasympathetic nervous system calms us when the stressor is gone, allows us to "rest and digest."

The body consistently demonstrates that it is more than just the mental chatter of the brain. We are not just consciousness living inside a body, we are our bodies. To separate our mind and emotions from the vessel that holds us and the spirit that enlivens us is a deadly mistake. Living in a body is not an abstract experience. However, after our socialization in Western culture, it takes a lot of convincing for people to commit to this.

Rene Descartes, an early European philosopher, proposed that thinking is the milestone of our existence. Because the information coming through our senses is so individual, we can trust it. His famous quote, "I think, therefore I am" was a huge contributor to our modern way of being. If I smell something foul and you don't, Descartes would say that we can't depend on our senses to give us objective information, so they never make us sure that we exist. Any indigenous person would likely conclude that was insane. To assume that humans or animals or plants do not exist because they don't think (or can't be proven to think) in the same way that other humans do is just not a reasonable conclusion. Our intellect grasps this easily. We dismiss Descartes as antiquated. Of course, we are not ignoring our bodies or treating them like objects. Yet, it is harder than that to undo centuries of habit that encourage us to live in our minds and ignore what our bodies say.

For years, I woke up and fed my dog. My white fuzzy dog and I developed this custom because she stood next to my bed, cleared her throat and nudged whatever parts of me that she could reach until I got out of bed. I let her out the back door to relieve herself and filled her bowl. I sat down for a few minutes to return phone calls, answer email and tackle my sinister hydra-like list of things to do. The next time I looked up, I had to go to work. I hadn't eaten and I inevitably had a slight headache and a nauseous feeling in my belly. Did my blood sugar drop or maybe it was mild dehydration? How did this happen again?

Why did I feed and take care of my dog reliably and not my own body? My body didn't urge me to care for it as strongly as my dog did. I convince myself of any number of excuses: I am just not hungry in the mornings, other things are more essential. I will grab something later in the day. My body endures choices for a long time and then suddenly, screams at me, Headache! Fatigue! Dizziness! Guess I'll have some more coffee.

Our bodies store memories, express emotion, and function (or not) according to our genetics, mood and life events. We can't reason with our bodies and if our bodies don't like the working conditions to which they are subjected, they will go on strike. We don't become ill because we are bad people. Poor health can arrive randomly or genetically, having it doesn't negate our inherent value and dignity. It is not a punishment.

Yet, sometimes illness demands that we pay attention to what is happening to us, to the decisions we make in our lives. Dr. Christiane Northrup says "You are not responsible for your illness; you are responsible to your illness." Health concerns demand that we make changes. The body participates in the conversation with the mind about shaping the reality that we experience.

In September of 2012, I stayed in a campground near the Breitenbush River in Oregon. At dusk, I wandered down the gravel road towards the dumpster to get rid of my trash. A movement on the side of the road captured my eye in the dim light. I made out the shape of a fairly large animal...a baby bear. I could not see a mother bear anywhere nearby. I buzzed all over, my body flashed quickly and then burned. A surge of energy persuaded me that I could run further and faster than any other animal. I grew three inches taller. Thought number one was "So, this is an adrenaline rush!" My second thought was "I've been wasting it on traffic and email!"

Adrenaline (Epinephrine) is a stress hormone secreted when we are under pressure to perform superhuman feats in a dangerous situation. The trouble is that we live in a culture that expects super-human feats daily. Many of us use caffeine to get ourselves out of bed and experience rushes of adrenaline sitting at computers, watching intense movies or navigating traffic. While the saying "mind over matter" may help us get through difficult conditions when we need to survive, "mind over matter" is not a sustainable way of life.

What would change if we could develop primary relationship with our bodies, if it were part of our spirituality? How might this change the ways we interact with other people or our own environment? Humans only recently live in situations where we do not interact regularly with the weather, food or our land base. I control the temperature of my home and travel in closed vehicles for my comfort.

In the urbanized world, we eat food that is wrapped in plastic and shipped over long distances. Sometimes, it does not look like the animal or plant from which it comes. This is convenient and sometimes less expensive, however, this makes food feel like a theory, available in aisles rather than a vital fuel source from the soil.

Every year, I bury the most petite tomato seeds in a pot on my porch. When the plant is knee high, I position the wire cage of three circles and cheer for those tiny yellow flowers to climb and produce the controversial fruit (or vegetable). If Portland doesn't get enough sun, sometimes they don't grow well, so I buy them at the Hollywood farmer's market. I know where my tomatoes come from. My body responds to the taste of them, their appearance, whether they are more delicious than last year. I know when the peaches come in four weeks late, or when the surprise March frost affects the cherries. I know what month that I can look forward to the blackberries, to the salmon, to the squash.

Eating seasonal foods provides the nutrients that help our bodies thrive within the cycles of the year. Great intelligence lies inside of native diets. The 'three sisters' of the American Southwest, corn, beans and tomatoes, grow together and lend nourishment to the traditional indigenous diet of that region. The restoration of native food ways is more than revolutionary, it is central. My body invests more in a place if I eat directly from that soil. Why then, is it normal to find highly processed food raised far away from my home and out of its growing season, especially at the markets in the transitional neighborhoods, far from Whole Foods. How are we to be healthy within a culture that acts in ways that are not?

It's time to hear spirituality speak through a body. Attention cultivates this doorway. The performance artist, Marina Abramovich mourns the loss of presence and attention in the modern age with *The Artist is Present*, a piece in which she sits in a table with two chairs. When the person sits down in a chair across from her, she is present with that person in silence. Intimacy builds. Discomfort appears. Tears arrive. People change their bodies in ways that are dramatic, shoulders drop, yawning sighs emerge. Others weep. With this exhibit, Abramovich provokes us to find attention and existence. We notice how far up the endangered list our presence inside our bodies and lives has already become.

Noticing the sensations that we are experiencing is a different way of living than the norm. Our minds easily distract us from feeling our clothes on our skin, our feet on the ground. Returning to those sensations can help us regain body awareness. When the sympathetic nervous system is activated, we often feel disassociated from our bodies. A focus on the sensations we feel right in that moment can restore us to present time. When I feel overwhelmed, and my body floats in space, I find three things I can hear or feel, even with my eyes closed. The better our practices are for returning to our own present moment, the more helpful we are to others who might be activated too. Our nervous systems naturally become attuned to each other as social animals. It is easy for someone with a relaxed nervous system to calm others in the room. With all the changes happening on the planet at this global moment, we definitely need calm nervous systems!

Chronic pain is a significant barrier to embodiment for people. I have acupuncture patients tell me that they do not enjoy being present when their bodies hurt. Studies often show that alongside medications, anti-inflammatory diets and physical therapy, some of the most effective pain relievers are breathing, herbs, meditation, acupuncture, heat/ice and gentle stretching. Changing our breathing habits affects pain levels and emotions. Breathing exercises can activate the vagus nerve, quiet adrenaline responses and slow down the heart.

Many cultures believe that breathing deeply can open us to connect with a greater source. There is a Dine/Navajo concept that the air inside of the lungs is contiguous with the air all around us. We all move through the same infinite, invisible, powerful medium. This connection provides a sense of shared spirit between humans and all breathing beings. This is another facet to Spirit that has been lost through the extreme individuation of Western urban culture. Inside our rugged loneliness, we live and work in very close quarters but we maintain our privacy by ignoring each other, pretending not to see the other bodies around us.

There are many practices that celebrate being a body: yoga, tai ch'i, qi gong, martial arts, dancing, sex, regular cardiovascular exercise and many more. These refocus our attention on the pleasure of moving or breathing into our bodies. Body-centered practices offer opportunities to experiment with what our bodies can actually do, not what our minds think they should be able to do. We now accept that people can be kinesthetic learners, what about the possibility of being kinesthetic worshippers?

Rabbi David Cooper founded a hybrid practice of Jewish and Buddhist meditation, affectionately referred to as BuJu. He tells us that "Every bodily movement has its source in the divine. Everything we do, everything seen or heard, tasted or touched, can be undertaken as a devotional practice." It is up to us to make sacred the experience of being our bodies. How could you offer your body more love and attention right now? When do you notice that you become disembodied? How frequent? How do you come back to the moment? Every minute we are alive, our hearts are beating, our lungs are breathing, and our blood is flowing.

Revolutionary Healing Dares:

I dare you to fall in love with your hard working body now, even before you lose the weight or stop the pain or the habit. Even before you change it in some way. I dare you to stand in front of the mirror naked and tell yourself "I love you" until you believe yourself saying it. I dare you to slow down and listen to the quiet voice of your body even if it tells you something else than what your mind wants to hear. I dare you to honor all of the bodies that you come in contact with as divine and plant the seeds for others to do the same.

Spiritual Inventory:
Exercises for Connection to Earth

Any sensing activity that assists people in developing self-awareness of their own bodies could be used for greater embodiment. These simple exercises are some of my personal favorites for my own grounding and centering. I also offer them to patients who have had good reasons to stay distracted from their bodily sensations, often those who have chronic pain or discomfort or who have experienced trauma. These exercises can be done separately or all together, depending on how much sensuality you would like to invite on any given day.

Before you begin, find a comfortable place to sit or lie down and take a few long slow breaths that fill every part of the lungs. A three-part breath that slowly fills the bottom, middle, and finally, the top of the lungs is very helpful.

1. **Breathing through the Senses:** The senses are gateways to the body's perception of reality, and spending some time with our awareness of what we perceive will increase our presence in our own bodily experience. Close your eyes. Inhale through the nose and imagine breathing out through the eyes. Open your eyes and notice several things that you see. Where are your eyes drawn? Inhale through the nose and breathe out through the ears. Take note of a few things you hear; try to listen beneath the obvious sounds. Close your eyes and breathe out through the pores of your skin, remembering that skin is the sense organ that covers the entire body. Become aware of at least two sensations of what is touching your skin; temperature of the air and weight of clothing count here! Breathe in and out through your nose and allow yourself to sniff deeply. What do you smell? Breathe in through your nose and out through your mouth and take in what you taste, you may notice if you are thirsty or hungry. Which sense is the most vivid? What are you noticing about your body today?

2. **Grounding:** Stand or sit with as erect a spine as possible. Feel the certainty of the bottoms of your feet on the floor or ground or perhaps your bottom in the seat. Visualize that your body becomes the trunk of a tree and you extend imaginary roots from the bottoms of your feet or the base of your spine into the floor or ground. Play with your weight, shifting from side to side if you are standing and shifting in a gentle circle around your spine if you are seated. Like a real tree, imagine water and nutrients rising through your trunk and the energy generated from this extending out your arms to your hands. Reach your arms overhead in a stretch as if they were branches. Many spiritual

and body-based traditions, like yoga, Qabalah, and European alchemy, have a practice of breathing up and down the spine from feet to head and back down to the feet. Let these breaths be effortless and circulate oxygen and energy throughout the whole body, picturing the breath going to every nook and crevice of the body. Sometimes it is great to mention specific parts of the body that we would not normally connect with the breath, like elbows, knees, fingertips, toes, behind the ears. These reminders can serve to help the breath go deeper and increase oxygenation of the whole system. If appropriate, it can be mentioned that trees and humans make a connection between the earth on which we stand and the heavens to which we look up and our spine can be a conduit between sky and ground.

3. I adapted this from Wendy Palmer, an aikido teacher in California, a three-part exercise from her aikido practice that she calls "**Attentional Concentration**." This exercise allows me to find myself home in my body with little effort.
a. Focus on the breath, particularly on a long exhale.
b. Play with balance and awareness to see if the weight of your body can be evenly distributed top to bottom and side to side.
c. Allow yourself to feel your actual weight and imagine all the mass of the atoms inside your body dropping to the bottom of those atoms.[1]

4. Self-massage: Begin with your hands and wrists and squeeze or massage them. You can massage up your arms to your neck and shoulders. You can press or rub your chest and work your way down your torso to the abdomen, gluts, legs, and feet. This can be very useful for reorienting to the body and tracking body sensation.

5. Felt Sense: This exercise is adapted from a technique developed by Gene Gendlin called the "felt sense." Tuning into our felt sense of circumstances in our lives can give us an awareness of how our body is feeling, which may or may not be the same as our mental or emotional state. The felt sense can teach us to speak the language of our bodies.

Give yourself a breath, pull your attention back from any external places, and let your eyes get soft or close them...

Imagine a situation in your life that you feel good about or perhaps a person who you really love or admire. Think about that person or situation, maybe recalling a memory or just a feeling of it or them. Notice how that feels in your body, where do you sense the feeling? How would you describe that feeling if you could? Does it have a quality that distinguishes it from other sensations in your body?

Imagine a situation that you have some conflicting emotions about. This could be a memory or just a feeling. What does that change in your body, where do you notice the feeling now? Does it have a quality, how is it different from the first sensation?

Some more questions to ask if you want to go deeper into the circumstances that feel challenging: What does this problem feel like? If I sense underneath the details, is there an impression that embraces this whole situation or person?

When you get an answer, it's great to ask, does this quality fit? What is it about this conflict that feels this way? Is there anything else for me to know?

It is great to sit quietly and to allow an answer to surface, to truly wait for the body to join the dialogue, expecting it to speak more slowly than the mind. Practice receiving whatever emerges from the position that your body speaking to you is a positive outcome.[2]

Living Inspiration: Jamie Seraphina Capranos

I spoke with Jamie Seraphina Capranos, a friend and colleague, about the concept of embodiment in medicine. She practices as a homeopathic physician and a midwife on Salt Spring Island, British Columbia, and travels throughout Canada and the US teaching herbalism courses to other practitioners.

GRS: Where do you personally see a hunger for the sacred the most?

JSC: I see that hunger in my medical practice. I work full time as a homeopath and midwife and a large percentage of my patients are between the ages of forty-five to sixty-five years old. Patients come in because they are having a crisis. Something about their physicality gets them in the door and asking for help, but we spend most of our time dealing with what you and I might call their underlying soul crisis. Many people come to Salt Spring Island to escape the grind of the city and live in a slower and more natural environment. At their stage in life, they have already given a lot to the world and, after all that they have given, they may be having a kind of existential crisis. They don't have the exact language for it, but they seem to want something more than work and family life. We often discover in our work together that they are craving an experience of the sacred.

I marvel at how few of us are taught this in all the places we are educated about the world: our families, schools, the media—how to bring some semblance of the sacred to our lives. I try to help people reconnect with their bodies. They are coming in with diagnoses of chronic pain or fibromyalgia for example, but they have no idea what is wrong. They are desperate for the symptoms to go away. Meanwhile, they are drinking twelve cups of coffee every day, they are hooked to their laptops, and when they take a break at all, they are eating white bread with margarine and mountains of sugar. They often do not understand the connection that is broken.

GRS: Where do you start?

JSC: I remind them that *we* are nature; our bodies are natural. In Chinese medicine, our physical functions change with the seasons. Our cardiovascular system alters depending on where the sun is in the sky; our bodies' needs change with the seasons. When I begin by just discussing processes that all humans share and our experience of a cycle of seasons, I'm able to enter the sacred with them without getting too "woo-woo." No one has to join a church or a spiritual group to bring back the rhythm of the life force that animates all beings. Everyone can relate to that rhythm; we all have a heartbeat.

I also see the hunger for the sacred in the school system around here. Whether it is young children or university students, people are subjected to a very mechanistic way of teaching. There is a real disregard for individual or even daily rhythms of people's bodies. Kids with ADHD or kids who are very empathic need something different than what the school system is providing. We need more education around different constitutions of bodies and how that applies to the way that we learn best, incorporate it into what we already know about differences in learning styles. What if we could understand ourselves as natural beings, and really try to connect to that pulse of nature in our decisions about learning? Learning itself could become a sacred practice, not a mechanistic task.

GRS: How did the concept of embodiment come to be a vital part of your life and work? Why is it of value to you?

JSC: I was raised by a mother who was a healer. From an early age, if we were ill, we went outside to heal in the sunshine, get fresh air. We got to run around with bare feet on the earth in the summertime, we built seasonal altars; this was a normal part of life. My grandparents were also herbalists so I grew up knowing that plants could heal our bodies when we became sick. I didn't realize how vital this was for me until I got older and engaged more with the wider world to see how much separation exists between humans and nature.

I was lucky to have gone through the Waldorf school system for my education, which helped me develop a trust in myself. Now, I see kids in that same school system playing outside with nature spirits, who they feel are their friends, developing confidence in their own opinions, in their own experience of the natural world. No one is telling them nature spirits don't exist; they will decide for themselves what is real about their relationship with the living earth as they get older.

GRS: Indigenous peoples all over the world believe that to say that to believe anything other than that the earth was alive was crazy.

JSC: Yes, and they would be right. Having an embodied practice must include a physical component and a way to connect to what is natural for human beings living on a planet that is also alive. The separation between mind and body is only two hundred years old. There was a time when everyone had basic access to medical information. It is profound for me as a practitioner to be with people who do not trust their bodies and need someone other than themselves to validate their experience. Sometimes people say, "When I eat dairy products, I get diarrhea. Should I stop eating dairy?" I see people who are over forty years old and do not know where their liver is or what their lymphatic system does. These are our bodies; it would be amazing if they were a little more familiar to us.

As I help to educate people about anatomy, and simple health practices, their confidence and personal responsibility for their own bodies increases dramatically. This kind of basic education about human bodies provided for all people could take a tremendous financial burden off of our health care systems. The Internet is doing some of this, but it helps to have another human to ask questions that are meaningful to you personally, to have someone with whom to interact.

As a teen, I sustained an injury to my spine that a whole lot of doctors declared untreatable and told me I would have a life of chronic pain. My mother took me to every kind of healer you can imagine but nothing worked to "cure" the pain. I began to take tai chi and hatha yoga classes even though at the time it was painful to move. Something about those practices helped me to trust the strength of my own body and to increase my own power, flexibility, and stability even while managing pain. It turns out that I needed to hear that I was strong from someone outside my family systems. In yoga classes, I was encouraged by my teachers to breathe into my own strength, the vital life force beyond pain. During one of my classes, I had an intuitive flash that whispered to me that I could heal myself, that it was possible to relieve my own pain.

Through my studies of homeopathy, I was able to do this. Even before I went to homeopathy school, my mom helped me find books about health and healing; we had long discussions together about what the pain could be telling me, teaching me. I really wanted to get the message! I realized during this time that our thoughts actually affect our physical health. I began to consider what could happen if I began to weed the unruly garden of my mind. I started a mindfulness practice which was life changing. I changed my mind, literally. With all of these things, my pain relief grew and I was able to return to more and more function. I was also happier, calmer, and much more embodied than I ever had been before my injury.

GRS: Why is homeopathy of value to you?

JSC: Homeopathy is the medical art of making sense of seemingly disparate symptoms. The things that seem insignificant to the patient are often vital information for the practitioners. It trains us to attend to details, and to listen to the body in a different way. Patients begin to pay attention over time that maybe digestion is connected to insomnia. This creates a picture we can see and a pattern we can track. Nothing is random; there is an inherent organization in the way the body creates illness, disorganizes tissue, why it produces a tumor at the exact site where it does. This is a very different perspective than the one we generally believe about the body!

As I journey in my own practice, there is a sense that nothing is accidental and a respect for the body's communication develops.

With the increase of this appreciation, there is a desire to know the body more deeply, to know the life force more intimately. It is quite simply the appreciation of the body's wisdom and the admiration of its intricacies.

GRS: Why is embodiment or this concept you present of finding a better or more intimate relationship with our bodies important to our collective health?

JSC: Embodiment is life promoting on any scale, personal or global. Cultivating a relationship with the life force within us is the ultimate way to honor, respect, and say yes to life, to live in the most vital way possible. Simply put, it fosters joy. We want this. When I think about it, I feel my cells smiling. It hasn't been scientifically proven yet, but I think it is on its way; we are studying happiness in more deliberate ways now. Creating a sense of embodiment and practicing it regularly is one of the greatest ways to combat anxiety and depression. As patients foster and develop a relationship with their own body and their own spirituality, their depression ameliorates. We need people on this earth who feel more alive, as this would inevitably lead to a more peaceful, generous, and loving society.

GRS: What are the side effects of a world where people don't value embodiment? What do you see as the major barriers to including these practices in the world we live in?

JSC: Humans are a microcosm; I am an expression of nature. In my medical practice, I see people harming themselves unconsciously through abuse of food, substances, and risky situations. They aren't even aware of causing themselves or other beings harm; this happens when we are disconnected. This harm extends to the earth: the way people poison their lawns with pesticides that end up in their neighbors' vegetable beds, the way people leave trucks running in parking lots, or clear-cut forests that provide habitat for animals, or get oil from the tar sands in northern Alberta. This is destruction but not for any kind of greater good, we are not destroying for a reason. We are living in anti-life, in an unconscious anti-life spell, and it is apparent on a large scale. These are all side effects of disembodiment.

One barrier to a practice of being present in our bodies is accessibility for people to whom this whole idea might be foreign. I work with folks that you and I might call very mainstream. If I get too abstract in the things I'm talking about, people can glaze over or look at me like I am crazy. As a more mature practitioner, I have learned that inaccessible language and abstract concepts are barriers. We have to give people a concrete reason to be here now, explaining why it is good in our pop-a-pill culture to listen to their bodies. As healers, we have to clarify exactly how being embodied will benefit you and make you feel good.

We are all emotional beings; even human beings who consider themselves very rational are constantly acting from an emotional place. People don't want to be given abstract rewards; no one can truly stay motivated toward living naturally because it brings something abstract like world peace. People want to hear what will make them feel good, sleep better, ease their constipation, and decrease their anxiety. We are interested in happiness.

GRS: It is a very different frame to consider that perhaps we as a species or a culture are trying to move to a place of ease, which is not always just self-serving.

JSC: Humans seek pleasure, sometimes by whatever means necessary! As a healer, I use that understanding as a tool. I remember working with a patient who was an investment banker who didn't know what I meant by the question, "What do you do for extracurricular fun?" He didn't have an answer. In these healing processes, we work on physical issues but we also work on the whole person. In this particular situation, part of my job as his practitioner was to ask him to find activities that he experiences as fun in the present moment and that inquiry has the potential to bring him home to his body. We have to learn how to literally speak to someone in their language, find a way into their whole psyche, and understand what they long for. That is what actually heals us.

GRS: What do you think would change in the world if placing a high value on embodiment became integrated in our culture or practices to cultivate embodiment became available within our systems of medicine?

JSC: I think that one piece of this solution is that it would take millions of dollars off our health care and welfare systems. This kind of treatment lasts longer, is more preventative, and leaves patients happier. Helping someone find their own form of embodiment is synonymous to helping someone tune in deeper to their purpose, not in a lofty sense, but in a very practical way. I have had patients who were gardeners and as they are deepening their embodiment practice, they decide hey, wait, I actually want to grow wildflowers, not garlic; through embodiment and the beginnings of self-awareness, people come into contact with their bliss. It can be practical, subtle, and profound. This is true not just in the example of the overworked doctor who drops out and becomes a violinist because that was her true bliss, but even in less dramatic changes, we can always see the benefit of people being able to tune in to themselves. Then they are able to notice: I want to turn my computer off at six p.m., because when I don't, it keeps me up all night. I think that folks having an internal silent check-in with themselves could be amazing. We have so little time, and we make so little time to just see what is going on inside ourselves. I would like to think we would see less violence, less pollution if people were willing to make the space for a little self-awareness.

GRS: What do you think would be altered if medical practitioners included the development of a sacred relationship with the body as an important factor in their recommendations for the treatment of illness?

JSC: I think it would be quite profound. Again, I think fewer drugs would be prescribed because the body wouldn't be shouting its symptoms in the same way. Our water supply would be incredibly altered if fewer medications were flushed into oceans and streams. Development of a relationship with our bodies would also be much cheaper than the kind of medicine we are currently practicing, suppressing symptoms so we can keep doing what we are doing. The impact of these practices on our personal and familial relationships would be amazing, like the twelve-year-old girl whose mother can now get out of bed because she no longer suffers from chronic fatigue syndrome because she is more aware of what happens when she gets overtired or she sees the connection between a gluten sensitivity and her energy levels and changes her diet for a while. We might have people who are happier and feeling more in alignment with their life's purpose. Humans are relational creatures, not solitary animals. We need each other. As one individual in a relationship becomes healthier and more embodied, it improves all the relationships that person has. People speak to each other more respectfully when they are present and in their bodies.

Ultimately, as romantic as it might sound, the effect of embodiment practices on a large scale becomes a happier nation making life-promoting decisions instead of death-promoting decisions. If medical practitioners could include the development of this kind of plan in all their treatment protocols, it might even inspire the healers themselves to have a more embodied practice. What if healers made time to care for themselves, paid attention to their own bodies? It would be a complete attitudinal shift; I liken it to a shift of axis point that would have a domino effect that we can't even begin to understand.

GRS: What is your offering to these interesting times in terms of your work? What does the world/what do humans need most right now in order to return to healthy culture?

JSC: I'm offering all the people I work with an opportunity to remember the conversation that is always going on with the mind and the body. We do this in a simple way, through using herbs and homeopathy and counseling, the medicines I use are clearing the obstacles between mind and body, creating a more unified holism.

I also offer the chance for people to appreciate that they are never alone in their despair. It is incredibly hard to break through the solitude because people feel so alone in their health problems, in their loss and suffering. Step one in this breakthrough would be accepting that even in the worst crisis, we are not alone. Most of us go through this disconnection or feeling of abandonment by a higher power at some point in our lives, or even at several points. Humans need most a deep empathy first for self and then for one another. We are united by our pain and also united in this journey of seeking joy even through the pain. We also need to learn to help each other. Returning to healthy culture includes sharing our experiences, ourselves, our ecstasy, our struggle, our wisdom, even with people who are not in our immediate circles.

I always come back to our involvement in the cycles of the seasons, of the natural world around us. We need to see our reflection in nature, not just as poetic and abstract but the practical applications that like many animals, we too need more sleep in the winter. As the plants die back, we might need to let go of extra responsibilities in the winter. We are made of the same life force and we can't ignore it any longer. The first step toward embodiment on a large scale and the kind of changes that would bring is for us to finally see that we are in fact, natural.

CHAPTER THREE

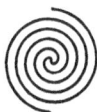

Connection to Earth:
The Living Web Around Us

...And no churches where God
is imprisoned and lamented
like a trapped and wounded animal.
The houses welcoming all who knock
and a sense of boundless offering
in all relations, and in you and me.
No yearning for an afterlife, no looking beyond,
no belittling of death,
but only longing for what belongs to us
and serving earth, lest we remain unused.

—RAINER MARIA RILKE

*A*t a spiritual retreat in the woods of Squamish, British Columbia, *we stand in a circle in a meadow among towering cedar and Douglas fir trees. One person asks out loud if the land will be our teacher. We pray to learn what it knows about what it needs, what it dreams of, how we can feed it and be fed by a relationship to it. Immedi-*

ately after the question is asked, a giant grey owl swoops overhead and we ooh and ahh as its silhouette is highlighted against the darkening sky.

∞

My patient comes to see me after camping for the first time after the end of her chemotherapy. Her face has a healthy color. Her pulses are steady and stronger than they have been in months. I ask her how the trip was and tears shine in her eyes, "I forget how much being out of doors can heal me." I offer her the assignment of listing the wild and beautiful places that she likes to go to in each season and then, committing to going there.

Sacred Exploration:

If establishing a relationship with our bodies answers the very important question of who we are, then establishing a connection to the land on which we live gives us a sense of where we are. We are human animals living within an ecosystem that supports us completely. Our divorce from any kind of practical reciprocity with land causes a kind of cognitive dissonance that we don't even know that we have. A healthy relationship to land base and a clear understanding of where resources come from has been an important component in many spiritual traditions. One might argue that this is paramount for the continued survival of a people and may certainly be a vital key to finding happiness.

What happens to make us believe that we are separate from our land base, that our actions don't have an effect on our environment? Joanna Macy, environmental activist and author, cites many reasons why people seem not to care. She believes we are afraid to feel the pain that might come with being connected to a planet that is in trouble. She goes on to say that we fear causing distress to others when we explain unpleasant truths about treatment of land by corporations, government, factory farmers. We may worry about experiencing guilt about not doing enough and not standing up for the places where we live. Macy suggests that the way past these fears is to open even more deeply, in community, to the truths we are facing as a species.[1]

Colonialists depicted native people as ignorant in order to justify the occupation of their land. The negative image of the dirty, uneducated, darker skinned, godless, dangerous savage held the projection of what settlers wanted to avoid at any cost. Another ideal was created, a superior archetype of civilization that allowed colonists to believe themselves to be clean, educated, white, religious, and nonviolent. For this ideal to thrive, the earth had to become "dirty" and living close to the land was equated with the worship of devils. This is reminiscent of the tactics used against the indigenous European healers to discredit them. Nearly every country in the world has been affected by European colonialism. Do we still live this way? Do we still want to live this way?

Spiritual customs of multiple native cultures involve the idea of conversation with their land base. Indigenous people constructed rituals for personal life events as well as to mark the change of seasons, ask for help and honor the beings with whom they share their home. Historians have said that this was proof of their ignorance, that to create rituals to celebrate the cyclical faces of nature was somehow antiquated. Science came along to "prove" there was no goddess of the moon, no songlines under the ground, no dance that could call the rain.

Spirituality is not a cerebral predicament. Just as prose exists without the attempt to replace poetry, so too can science live alongside of ritual and art. When we lose this kind of poetry, we also let go of a trust in place, or any relationship in which we wonder what the other being needs and wants. Connection to land may ask us to find a kind of indigenous trust in our relationship to the earth.

There is something that happens when we have encounters with wild nature that makes us feel more fundamentally human. There are parks, nature centers, and protected lands all over the globe designed to preserve and protect wild earth. We seem to enjoy "vacationing" there to restore our mental health; the ocean, the mountains, the rivers and lakes, the desert, the forest have become destinations for us. We are beginning to understand that these places are connected to our physical health and to make connections between deforestation and flooding or between factory waste and our watersheds.

We may understand that we can't live without these refuges but can we expand to include them in our idea of where we do live? We need to believe that we have a place on this planet, that our idea of home is bigger than a house or apartment number on an urban street. Many have argued that a large-scale reanimation of this belief would change the way we interact with our planet's resources.

If many more of the earth's modern human inhabitants began to find some aspect of our spirituality rooted in the land, we might stop spraying poison on our food, permitting chemicals to permeate our water, hunting species to extinction. We might find the courage to stand up even more firmly to the entities that continue to support these behaviors. If we began to have conversations with the earth again, perhaps the earth would gain a voice in our governments' decisions and would be considered as we develop madly toward covering every inch of the planet with more roads, structures, and concrete.

Leading the world in environmental lawmaking, Bolivia drafted eleven rights for nature, called the Law of the Rights of Mother Earth. These include the earth's right to life and to exist; the right to continue vital cycles and processes free from human alteration; the right to pure water and clean air; the right to balance; the right not to be polluted; and the right to not have cellular structures modified or genetically altered. With experimental wording that will surely challenge the mining industry of Bolivia for years to come, these laws also describe the right of nature "to not be affected by mega-infrastructure and development projects that affect the balance of ecosystems and the local inhabitant communities." In April of 2011, Bolivian Vice President Álvaro García Linera said, "It makes world history. Earth is the mother of all. It establishes a new relationship between man and nature, the harmony of which must be preserved as a guarantee of its regeneration."[2] What will have to change in the minds of policymakers in the Western world to believe that listening to and considering the land in decision making is not only sane but desperately needed for our health?

There are accounts that human languages were developed from the calls of birds and the noises of animals.[3] Joining into the conversation around them, ancient humans may have developed language that blended into the landscape, which reaffirmed them as a part of the ecosystem rather than separate from it. In this theory, different landscapes and ecosystems would produce vastly different languages for the beings that lived there. This would make the conversation between people and land something beyond a metaphor.

Stephen Harrod Buhner, herbalist and author, says that encounters with wild nature create something irreplaceable in humans, an experience that is necessary to our health. This "something" may not happen if we are only interacting with other humans and domesticated animals. Anyone who has ever seen a wild animal outside a zoo can probably identify with this statement. Looking into the eyes of another being feels primal.[4] Even many hunters often describe this as a sacred moment, particularly those who hunt for food rather than sport. I believe that what happens in these moments is an affirmation of the truth that we are not alone on the planet, not the only conscious species. Even our affection for our pets is an echo of this bond. Many studies have shown that connecting with a pet reduces stress and increases health benefits. Why do we share pictures of cute animals with each other on the internet? Something awakens in us when we see these friends of ours.

What connection do you have to the land on which you live? Where do you feel related to the planet? Are there beautiful or special places that you visit regularly? What actions can you take for the health care of the land where you live? This might become an important prescription for your health care.

As an acupuncturist, I have prescribed food from the closest farmer's market for many of my patients, sometimes asking them to purchase local honey or leafy greens. I give them recipes to try an anti-inflammatory cleansing diet for thirty days. I have asked people with knee injuries to stop running on concrete and given them trail maps for many of the gorgeous hiking trails around Portland. For many people, gardening is part of a remedy for depression or grief.

Returning to some version of this interdependence with land is a threshold for us to cross in our relationship to health care. It can truly be this simple to return to our health, our home, ourselves.

Revolutionary Healing Dares:

I dare you to look up your favorite animal, where it lives and what is happening with its health and habitat right now. I dare you to do one thing to help them thrive. I dare you to go to the places that are so beautiful that you could cry. I dare you to allow yourself to care about them as much as you do your family and friends and share them with the people you love. I dare you to clean them up, to protect them, to ask them and get to know what they need. I dare you to ask other people about their sacred places and what makes those places precious. If these places do not spring quickly to your mind, perhaps it is time to go in search of them.

Spiritual Inventory:
Exercises for Connection to Earth

1. Make a list of ten native plants that grow in your area. Purchase a plant guide or check one out from the library to learn to identify them and some lesser known facts about them. Where do they like to grow? What time of year do they bloom? Are they edible or do they have any medicinal uses? Go on a hike or a plant, herb, or mushroom walk being offered by a nature society in your area and practice finding them.

2. Find the nearest farmer's market in your area and make it a point to go there. Look for your favorite fruits and vegetables and see what other foods are raised or made locally. What grows in each season where you live? What are the treats that spring, summer, and fall bring?

3. This is an exercise adapted from *The Earth Path* by Starhawk that helps us practice consistent inquiry into what is going on with the plants and animals around us. Select an outside location in which to sit regularly and just watch what is going on around you. This can be your backyard or a park nearby, somewhere that feels like a place where you can watch birds and other animals going about their lives. Schedule times to go and sit there for fifteen to twenty minutes, being as unobtrusive as possible. Daily observation is a great goal but even once or a few times a week can work. Look for repeated patterns: Where are the birds' favorite trees? Where do the squirrels or other animals live? Why do certain plants grow together? What are their names? It is great to ask yourself questions about why certain things that you witness happen and then either look up the information or ask people you know. Your research will become a great conversation starter [5].

Living Inspiration: Starhawk

Starhawk is a visionary author of many books, including the novel *The Fifth Sacred Thing*. She is also a longtime peace and earth activist, voice of Goddess religion, and permaculture teacher who lives in the San Francisco Bay Area and teaches internationally. I met with Starhawk in Molalla, Oregon, at a spiritual retreat to talk about human relationship to land base.

GRS: Where do you personally see a hunger for the sacred the most?

S: Right now, I see it in young people. Where I see the hunger for the sacred, for wonder, has shifted a lot in the last couple of years. Sometimes I am invited to speak at music festivals. Three or four years ago, I was invited to give a talk and lead a ritual at a large music festival and thirty people showed up to participate. Last year at the Symbiosis festival, over a thousand people attended the talk and spiral dance and they wanted to know more, how they could continue finding spiritual practices in their own lives. A lot of the energy that we see people invest in the use of drugs and alcohol is a deep hunger for spiritual experience.

These days, I teach permaculture a lot. I see the same hunger for the sacred in the people attracted to permaculture and people attracted to do some kind of meaningful work with the earth. People want their hands in the soil, to garden and grow food in ways that heal and support the land that is always there all around them. In our two weeklong Earth Activist Trainings, we teach people permaculture as a form of activism. We start with permaculture as the foundation and then extend the principles and insights of permaculture into progressive political organizing, and explore strategies for change. We weave in threads of Earth-based spirituality, inclusive and nondogmatic, to connect heart and soul to the work. We always add nature awareness as the touchstone. Our Earth Activist Training offers a rich array of solutions, tools, and strategies to redesign our world.

GRS: Will you say more about permaculture and how you see its role in the larger healing process for the planet?

S: "Permaculture" is regenerative design: a set of ethics, principles, and practices that create beneficial relationships and whole systems. Permaculture meets human needs sustainably and heals damaged natural systems. Permaculture works with nature, or rather, teaches us to act in the same way we see nature working, rather than fight against natural processes.

I often teach in the inner city, so I see the hunger for spiritual experience in folks who have a relationship with public housing and criminal justice. It is hard to bring in spirituality to those situations but I do see that longing for the sacred in them. We create gardens together in public spaces or in schoolyards and we have a lot of conversations while we are working. Talking to people about what really matters to them, what is important, asking them where in their lives they feel they can make a difference really speaks to them in a way that simply asking them to eat their veggies because it's good for their health does not.

One of my projects right now is making a movie out of my novel, *The Fifth Sacred Thing*. In Hollywood, even among people who are very successful, there is a subculture of people very hungry for the sacred. I have come across entire organizations dedicated to figuring out how to bring those practices into making movies. It was quite surprising to discover how passionately people feel about this in the movie industry.

GRS: How did a connection to land come to be a vital part of your life and work? Why is it of value to you?

S: I've always loved nature and loved gardening. That was always a big part of Goddess and Earth-based religion, that nature is sacred. As part of that, I began studying permaculture in the late 1980s and early '90s. I was fortunate enough to get land of my own so I could experience living and working over time with a piece of land. Living and building relationship with the same land over time deepened my sense that spirit and the sacred are connected to how we bond to and make a commitment to a place. The land is a place where my energy gets renewed. It is the basis of life. We absolutely cannot live without it. We have to get food and water from somewhere, and the ecosystems around us are what sustain our life, all life.

GRS: Do you ever find people surprised by that?

S: A lot of people in Western culture are completely disconnected from nature. Kids in our inner city permaculture program say to us, "We can't eat the shit that grew in the garden, that was in the dirt." People think soil is "dirty," rather than life giving. There are a lot of people for whom spirit is about removal from nature, about the disconnection, about transcending the physical plane in which we live.

GRS: Why is a connection to our land base important to our collective health?

S: If we are not connected to the land, and we don't take care of the land, we're not going to eat, have water to drink, clean air to breathe. If you grow food in soil where you have already built soil structure that is full of vitality and minerals, when you eat that food you have a wildly different experience than eating food wrapped in plastic that we buy at the grocery store out of its growing season. Our physical health depends on the land; we are definitely not getting the nutrition we are supposed to get from food that is devitalized, shipped all over world, and sprayed with chemicals. The health of food depends on the health of the soil and our health depends on the health of food. We are quite literally dependent on the soil for our health. The more of us who understand this, the better. We can begin to purposefully heal and enrich our soil, knowing that we are reliant upon its vitality and minerals.

GRS: What are the side effects of a world where people don't value relationship to the earth?

S: I think we are seeing side effects in the ways that we don't value interconnectedness. We see ourselves as separate from the natural world. We are rapidly destroying basic life support systems because we don't see that we are an integral part of them or at least deeply affected by them. Climate change is progressing at a high rate. Our current economic system values short-term profits and doesn't value the life-support systems of the planet. This is a disastrous way of thinking.

GRS: What do you see as the major barriers to including these practices in the world we live in?

S: Some of the barriers are that society as a whole doesn't value or teach connection to the land, and people have to seek it outside of typical education systems. Some of the barriers are internal. With young people, what's hip and cool is not about the land. It's hard to get young people excited about growing food and doing things like digging, weeding, planting that are hard physical work! Although that isn't always true; many of our permaculture classes are full of young, white, middle-class youth eager to get out with shovels. However, kids who come out of poverty, who don't have yards or families who garden, they often don't want to get dirty. It's sometimes much harder to get them motivated to kneel in the soil. In the schools, we've seen it's important for social status to wear snow-white tennis shoes that no one wants to get muddy. And it's popular for many of the girls to have beautifully manicured nails, which can certainly be an obstacle to gardening! Many of the things in the culture that are marks of self-esteem or respect are marks against getting closer to the earth. Little kids like to play in the dirt, play with the bugs. They are completely fascinated by it if you get them young enough. That curiosity tends to wane as kids get older.

In one permaculture project, we built a container garden on an asphalt lot that surrounds many offices and their new office was in the housing projects. It was in a cement block building that had been refurbished to house these offices. We ran a permaculture program and built an entire garden. A gang of ten-year-olds got into the building and vandalized it. People in the neighborhood did some work with them and even some of their older brothers had talks with them and told them, "You can't do that stuff around here, because this is my job." The message hit home; the garden and the office belonged to the neighborhood. Now the kids jump over the fence and water our plants.

GRS: What changed their minds?

S: Community pressure was a big factor. After the community talked with them, the kids came in a couple of times and everyone on the project also talked to them, made them feel welcome, and helped them get involved. It turns out that one little boy loves to garden, he told me that he has his own garden at home, so I gave him some plants from the garden. He is a larger little boy, and couldn't get over the fence easily like the others. I identified with him and threw him a bucket to help him climb the fence. He became even more curious about what we were doing and has stayed interested.

GRS: What do you think would change in the world if a more personal connection to land became integrated in our culture or available within our systems of medicine? For instance, what would be altered if medical practitioners included the development of a relationship with the natural world as an important factor in their recommendations for the treatment of illness?

S: We would have a holistic approach to medicine and healing if people were encouraged to grow and eat their own food grown in living healthy soil and we were able to prioritize practices to keep the soil that healthy. We would see more integration of physical and spiritual health. There is so much sickness right now—cancers, autoimmune disorders, severe food allergies. It has to be related to the sickness of earth, the toxins of cities, to the terrible food that most people eat.

GRS: Most healers tear their hair out trying to figure out what to do to help people when we suspect the environment itself is making us sick. If we could learn to heal and change on that level, we might have a shot.

S: My own health drastically improved since we got land and I started spending time outside. If you are putting out a lot of effort and working really hard, you need connection to vital energy that is present in the forest and the ocean. These subtle energies are important to keep our energy alive and vibrant.

At one point I noticed that I knew so many people who had autoimmune disorders. I also used to get completely exhausted and worried that might be happening to me. When I started spending regular time outside on the same piece of land, it really shifted for me. My energy was rejuvenated by that time, and my body was healed by that relationship.

GRS: What is your offering to these interesting times in terms of your work?

S: My work these days is about telling stories that hopefully can warn and inspire people to look at the world differently. I am also teaching people the skills of connection, community building, and permaculture, all vital to our continued existence on the planet.

GRS: What does the world/what do humans need most right now in order to return to healthy culture?

S: I think we need a deep shift in values from a world that values objects and profit to a world that values relationships to the earth, each other, plants and animals. The whole world is basically a network of relationships.

I think we are in a time of tremendous loss. Some losses we already know we are on the verge of experiencing. For the sake of our collective health, we have to learn to deal with loss and grief and still do whatever we can to save, conserve, and protect what we can. We must learn a lot about building resiliency.

GRS: Yes, it seems that we are continuously getting lessons about how to keep going when it seems hopeless. Can you speak more about resiliency?

S: The transition town movement talks about the idea that a community can develop resources that allow it to bounce back after catastrophe or setback. On a community level, that is all about having local food systems, healing systems, and knowing where clean water comes from. It's about having multiple ways of meeting our needs, creating and sustaining local production and industries, rather than depending on large corporations. Resilience is about building networks where people take care of one another. We can recover from anything if we are well networked.

CHAPTER FOUR

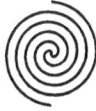

Ritual: When We Create Sacred Space

loneliness does not make sense
when there are so very many of us
bumping hollow shells and murmuring empty
pardons and apologies. do we waste our days...
saying we seek to understand the why of it
i must stop believing there is space at all
between you and me when i feel the fear
of our hearts shuddering as one.

— SARWAT RUMI

For a week or more in the summer of 2001, fires burn through northern New Mexico forests in the Pecos Wilderness and Los Alamos, creating thick gray smoke that threatens animals in the forests and people in Santa Fe. People have to evacuate their homes and firefighters are battling the flames day and night. No one knows when the monsoon season will begin. My friends from Santa Fe come to stay in Albuquerque to escape the smoke. We gather in the backyard of my friend's house and drum and sing songs about rain, dance for rain, express our longing for rain in every language we know. We know that *we don't have any idea how to call the clouds or if it is even possible to conjure rain, but we ask the skies for help as plainly as we can for all the beings in danger from the encroaching fires. At the end of the ritual, we acknowledge to each other that we feel more hopeful if nothing else, less desperate about the dryness. A few days later, I stand in the checkout line at the La Montanita Co-op and someone bursts into the store and announces, "It's raining!" Everyone leaves their position in line, even the cashiers, and we all pour out of the doors and turn our faces up to the falling rain.*

A patient is having difficulty conceiving even though all her tests come back normal. We talk and she tells me that she had an abortion when she was very young and still feels guilty about this decision even though she knows it was the right one for her. We talk about what the body might believe that the rational parts of ourselves do not and about the power of ritual to get all parts of us on the same page. She decides to do a ritual to honor the baby that was lost and comfort herself for making that choice. We think of ways she could use ritual to communicate with her body, mind, and spirit that she is ready to have another child now, times have really changed, and now it is safe. She decides to ask her friends to help her by offering her fertility blessings and prayers.

Sacred Exploration:

Ritual is essential to the world right now. A crucial part of the revolutionary healing of our world is to invite the design and practice of rituals back into our lives. Ritual gives us the audacity to believe that we can change events in our lives and our communities. The practice of ritual endows us with more opportunities to get out of our heads, into our bodies, and connected to the earth.

Our bodies respond to ritual. Our connection to land has traditionally inspired humans to create ritual to celebrate cycles of seasons and the flora and fauna with whom we are interdependent. For many cultures, this has been the foundation of their spirituality and often, their collective health. The archetype of ritual answers the question of how we draw together bodies and land and time. Ritual has the ability to connect people over great distances and centuries.

A familial connection to land traditionally inspired humans to create ritual to celebrate cycles of seasons and the flora and fauna with whom we are interdependent. For many cultures, this became the foundation of spirituality and often, collective health. Ritual heals, marks the passing of cycles, celebrates, changes something, or offers prayers for an outcome.

When we step into a ritual space, we relax the logistical left brain way of thinking and enter the right brain imagination and sensuality. We enter the timeless realms, the world where mythology, poetry, divine beings and archetypes live and breathe. Ritual takes place outside of clock time. It is one of the few places where we unfetter the creative brain and allow it to play. In ritual, the impossible becomes possible. We are not held back by the same rules of order that exist in our linear and formed ways of life. Ritual can be simple or elaborate. Ritual can remind us that the world is more mysterious and unpredictable than we believe.

Albert Einstein said, "The most beautiful thing we can experience is the mysterious. It is the source of all true art and all science." The truth is that we may need mysterious experiences like this to remain psychologically sound, trying on the idea of a vast pattern in which we are held. Ritual reminds us of the unity that exists beneath the surface of the illusion that everything is divided into compartmentalized objects. Many religious traditions and spiritual paths base themselves in a belief that we are threads of an immense tapestry that is reality. Science, especially quantum physics, continues to discover that many of the spiritual beliefs around unity are indeed correct on a subatomic level. Ritual often gives us this sensation of being connected to all things.

A ritual is usually marked by our entering into a state of being that is qualitatively different than our everyday way of being or thinking. We might call this sacred space because it asks us to change our consciousness and attention in order to be present. Some cultures have made it an art form in and of itself. The creation of ritual that speaks to us is the talent of the ritual artist. Modern theater performance has its roots in ancient rituals.

Other times, the repetition of the ritual is what holds the sacred. The very fact that the ritual has been performed so many times causes us to give it more relevance or reverence. This practice links us to the people who lived before us over great distances and centuries. Lighting the menorah on Chanukah makes bonds with ancestors who have ignited candles in this same way for centuries to celebrate the miracle of the oil.

Ritual is meant to touch us at a deep level, though our logical minds may not understand what is happening. The body and our primal selves respond to symbol, rhythm, song, movement, play. Children build rituals instinctually without knowing exactly what they are doing. We construct ritual in our daily lives around transitions, almost unconsciously. Brewing our first cup of coffee in the morning, greeting our family when we arrive home for the day. We dismiss them as meaningless routines, but the truth is that they hold great import for us and are difficult to change. Sometimes a change in our rituals evokes intense emotions because we are so invested in them. A familiar form of ritual in the Western world is the bedtime routine, often including some kind of prayer or gratitude for the day. We prepare the conscious mind to turn inward, stating intentions and asking for help. Asking to connect with the divine or with an intention to end the day is an act that holds power.

Many modern holidays have become commercialized and non-representational so they do not have the function to remind us of what is happening right now in our ecosystems. Enacting ritual has the potential to connect us to the land on which we live, but also to our own bodies and each other. When ritual is taken out of the context of living on land in present time in human bodies, it becomes abstract. We forget why ritual ever had value or vitality.

The collective movement away from ritual in our modern culture bases itself on the accusation that practicing rituals was silly, dangerous or primitive. Primitive is exactly what ritual may be, in terms of accessing our subconscious. We can't measure exactly how much impact our subconscious mind has on our behavior, but we know it is a factor. It is often a surprise to examine what we hold to be true at a deeper level that does not register in our conscious experience. It may be only in the more subterranean parts of ourselves that we can release the rigid hold we have on our false beliefs, habits, and addictions.

Often, we strive to change behavior we may have outgrown or patterns that do not serve us any longer, on a personal or communal level. This kind of transformation requires more than just our mental acuity. These are not intellectual problems and no matter how much we attempt to reason with ourselves, we don't usually shift our actions as a result of giving ourselves a good talking-to. Ritual opens a window into the parts of our body, mind and spirit that are more ancient, anchored in the deepest reserves of the brain and heart.

There are so many times that we desperately hope to change ourselves or another's consciousness or behavior. Sometimes we can hold very strong opinions about what we "should" be doing instead and still do not change our behavior. Because it works on more than one level, ritual can facilitate this complete shift in consciousness.

We cannot change our patterns of behavior through logic alone. This practice takes more than just thinking positively. In ritual, our reality expands to include symbolism, art, and imagery as valuable communication. Our right brain hemisphere comes into play, the part of us that responds to mythology and imagination, which can see beyond current circumstances. We are able to recognize metaphor, archetype, and timelessness. We can open to solutions and ideas that are beyond list-making, will power and details.

Sensory input from living in cities places stress on our nervous systems even without our awareness. Ritual creates separate space and time to set all the excess stimulation in our lives aside. It allows for the expression of gratitude, to recognize what is sacred around us. A student of mine once pointed out that most indigenous practice is a continued expression of gratitude. In modern civilization, we sometimes believe that we can have what we want without giving thanks or reciprocity. Consumer culture is the opposite of gratitude, it often keeps us in "I want it now and I want more of it." Neurochemistry tells us that gratitude interrupts negative thought patterns in the brain and changes emotional states, which is all the more reason to reinvigorate gratitude rituals.

It is radical to give sacred space a central role in our lives, to say that this is the essence of what is most important. It is revolutionary to express ourselves, to be creative and explore our own spiritual values through the design of ritual. It can feel risky to defy the fears that we will be dismissed or denigrated as modern humans if we craft rituals. It is challenging to move past the part of ourselves that tells us that ritual is ridiculous, or that it doesn't work. There are also ideas left over from colonization and the erasure of indigenous peoples that we will be harmed somehow if we venture outside of the box that has been made for us.

We are beginning to realize the need for ritual is contemporary and relevant to our health. Humans need to touch infinite spaces, to designate time for the visionary. Even the brainstorm sessions that we do in workplace meetings are a type of ritual. We are in a time of transition from what has been to what could be and ritual helps us connect to past, present, and future. Whether about individual journeys or our collective future, ritual is a powerful visioning tool that imparts insight about what we want to come of this changing time.

Revolutionary Healing Dares:

I dare you to create ritual for your modern life. I dare you to step between the world that does not believe in magic and mystery and the world that does. I dare you to pay homage to what is sacred about your life in this non-ordinary place in some creative way. I dare you to perform rituals that celebrate and rebuild your personal health and our collective health care and ask other people to help you and help themselves.

I dare you to ask for the changes you want to see on this planet that we share and use ritual as yet another way to bring them into being.

Spiritual Inventory:
Exercises for Ritual Creation

1. **Calendar therapy:** Set aside specific sacred space in your life. What times could you set aside in your life for ritual? Do you need this on a daily basis or perhaps to mark a particular upcoming or recently past transition? Sit down with your calendar and mark out short or longer periods of time that you hold aside for honoring what is happening in your life with a ritual. This could be the fifteen minutes after the kids go to bed to make a list of what you are grateful for or the hour before you have to be at work for a home yoga practice focused on an intention that you choose. If it is a particularly significant or challenging time in your life, you can set aside more time to do a more involved ritual that illustrates or attends to that particular situation as well.

2. **Journal writing:** Sit down with your journal or a blank piece of

paper. How do you or would you create sacred space for yourself or others? What qualities or items in a space really change it from mundane to special? What kinds of words or language change the quality of an environment from linear to more timeless? Make a list of ways that you make a space or an event more precious or momentous. Do you decorate, light a candle, play music? How might that apply to creating ritual space?

3. **Ritual design:** You have decided to create some kind of a personal ritual. Here are some things to consider to make it effective:

- What situation is calling for a ritual?
- What is it that you want to communicate within the ritual, what is the core?
- What is the intention that you would like this ritual to hold or the energy you would like to transform?
- What is the emotional content with which you want to work?
- Is there space for some kind of creative activity?
- What items or logistical space and time do you need in order to do the ritual?
- Is there room for something mysterious or unplanned to happen inside it?
- What outcome are you looking for? [1]

4. **Simple ritual experiment:** Light a candle and sit in stillness for a few moments, taking long slow breaths into all parts of your lungs. Do a short meditation on the difficulties in your life that you would like to release, or change your emotional attachment to. Write on a piece of paper these situations or circumstances. You can choose whether to burn it, tear it up into pieces and put it into the compost, bury it, or dissolve this paper in water. Write on another piece of paper a list of things that you are grateful for. You can decorate it any way you like; hold onto this piece of paper, post it somewhere you can see it frequently. When this is complete, blow out the candle and notice how you feel. Has anything shifted for you? What about after a few days?

5. Tracking rituals that already exist: Do your family or friends

have any seasonal or regular rituals? Do you and your partner or lover have special rituals that have meaning for you? What do you do for birthdays and other holidays? How do you celebrate when something great happens? How do you support each other when a really challenging event happens? How do you mark loss or change? If some of these things seem pertinent, you might contact some folks in your life and ask them what they have done or would like to do when these kinds of life events happen. Brainstorm about possibilities for rituals and share them among yourselves. Discuss rituals that you would like to have or do in the future.

Living Inspiration: Suzanne Sterling

Suzanne Sterling is a phenomenal musician, educator, and cofounder of a nonprofit called Off the Mat, Into the World. Through Off the Mat, she helps to raise funds for third world community projects and travels internationally to bring those projects to life. I have worked with Suzanne on a number of collaborations involving art, mythology, music, spirituality, and healing and consider her a true ritual artisan. We discussed the importance of ritual in healing practices in the Mission District of San Francisco.

GRS: Where do you personally see a hunger for the sacred the most?

SS: I see it in almost all of the people that I encounter in workshops across the country and in personal situations. They are having so much disillusionment with our pop culture or the way their lives intertwine with pop culture, by which I mean the distractions and underlying dissatisfaction of what is, primarily, Western culture. There is a longing to connect to the immortal that lives in us. I see it in our culture's interest in myth, ritual, sexuality, and magic, and the simultaneous fear of it. I see the most hunger in Western culture or dominant culture. There is a great challenge as developing countries are trying to meet up with Western culture in terms of material goods and technological advances. There is a way in which they are willing to (or being forced to) throw out the value and meaning of their indigenous culture in an effort to chase the material security and the power that comes with that, that is evident in Western culture. For me some of the most interesting places I have been are where I've seen indigenous culture meet Western culture. I have seen that there is still a connection to earth, self-expression, soul, nature, and spirituality, even if it has been turned into a Westernized version of itself. These are still strong and present in many cultures all over the world. However, in the West, people have lost a sense of the sacred and their own personal relationship to the sacred. A byproduct of this is a loss of their own self-expression and an inherent right to their own artistry.

GRS: Can you speak a little bit about the cultures that you feel still have this unbroken connection to soul, nature, and spirit?

SS: I've now traveled to Cambodia, Uganda, Haiti, India, and South Africa. Especially in the smaller villages where I have visited, there is a sense of immediacy around living with land, song and dance, self-expression and ritual. It is deeply inherent; there is not even a question about being able to create art, song, or ritual. As someone who comes and brings Westerners to these places, I have noticed surprise in the people who live there when we are willing to interact. People often sing to us when we visit and they are always surprised when the groups we take to these places sing back to them. To me, this sort of expressive exchange is natural so that surprise is a sad statement about our dominant culture.

I spend a lot of time working in the yoga world and I see the yoga practice as a portal into spirituality. What I love about the yoga practice is that it brings us even more into our bodies and reminds us that we can have a more intense embodied life. In a serious yoga practice, the grip of consumerism loosens. The grip of the rat race, self-hatred, and self-criticism loosens, the meaning of consuming for the sake of consumption, or to feel better, comes into question. Then there is this moment, where we say, if I am not here just to consume, okay, what is next? People don't often have a context to create what is next. They don't know what is missing; they only feel emptied out. They don't really care to have the next great car, the large house, the next great set of clothes. In fact, that level of ownership of things is very complicated. They begin to participate in a simplification of their lives, perhaps a release from drugs/alcohol, and a sense develops of wanting to be part of the solution. They may find a personal spirituality. Yoga can do that but there are many different forms of yoga and people aren't always being spoken to at the deepest level in their yoga practice. They just become aware in the silences that there is something more. They know that their traditional forms of spirituality somehow don't cut it. Developing a purely traditional form of yogic philosophy doesn't always work for our modern day language either. That is where I come in. Much of my work is to help people figure out what it is that moves them about ancient practices, how they can augment these practices. How is it applicable to their day-to-day lives? For a lot of people it means being of service. That is their spirituality in action. They may not know exactly how to do that and that is the next step for a lot of people.

GRS: How did ritual come to be a vital part of your life and work? Why is it of value to you?

SS: That is a hard question to answer. It's been a part of my life for so long. The initiation of my work with ritual came from inside of me as a reaction to my challenging childhood and a sense that there were more layers of perception than I could articulate, but felt deeply in my bones. I had some amazing teachers early on who helped to connect me with worldwide spiritual practices and nature-based awareness. Some of my early teachers helped me to create a spiritual context for everything I did. Slowly, that grew over time to become my life's work. From a very early age, I have had one foot in the mythological world, one foot in the practical world. My training as a ritualist has been trying to bridge worlds as much as possible in a way that is accessible for other people.

Personally I'm a rationalist so it's important for me to not get lost in my own critical thinking or just the doing of things and step into a deeper life of meaning and purpose. I also found connection with Spirit through art for a long time and that has continued to be the case. My art has been an expression of my spiritual connection but now it is more than that. I'm starting to see that at a practical, cultural level, my work can give voice to that bridging between the worlds. That is what ritual does.

If I personally get far away from my own daily practice or my personal rituals, I can get aggravated, angry, frustrated and feel a lack of meaning in life. The separation from ritual doesn't serve me. Art and ritual ask me to make the harder choice to step into risk and continue to evolve. That choice to not take the easy or secure route is not a choice that everyone is willing to make.

In comfort, people stop growing. People grow because they are challenged and meet the challenge with the best part of themselves. When we open to lives that are a little out of our comfort zone, it keeps us alive and healthy. Nature is not comfortable, but modern civilization has tricked us into thinking that our lives should be comfortable so we have lost touch with both the power and the danger of nature. And yet, this is a place where we can find growth, inspiration, and wisdom.

GRS: Why is the concept of ritual important to our collective health?

SS: My favorite expression is that ritual is "finding soul expression in community"; soul expression is an inherent human right. I believe that everyone wants to find their inner artists. This may not be an artist who gets paid for what they do or who deals with the pressures of an artistic career. Rather I am talking about permission for a self-expression that is not rational, that doesn't have to make sense...a self-expression that is mythological, beyond our human comprehension, and drops us into the mystery of things.

Ritual has a mythological context. In community, expressing ourselves at this level changes us, and this personal expression is one of the healthiest things we can do. If I speak about it in terms of singing, what happens when people want to sing and their voices get shut down, as often happens in a childhood of trauma or intense criticism or abuse? The results of this are that the vibratory expressive system goes into shutdown to protect us...it goes into inertia. This kind of protective shutting down/inertia over time can quite literally cause disease. In both nature and in humans, when energy is not alive and vibrating, i.e., moving, systems become unhealthy. When people allow themselves to express—using their voices, bodies, or emotions—the flow of life force (or chi or energy) does not get stuck in the body, and the system automatically heals itself!

In ritual we find a kind of "collective healing" by going into what is called "sympathetic resonance" with each other and reaching states of consciousness that are transformative on a collective level. On a brain level, we literally have an experience of oneness when we go into sympathetic resonance together. Experiencing these altered states of consciousness or perhaps the kind of consciousness that lives just beneath the normal waking state, brings all parts of our brain online, shuts down the dominance of the neocortex a little bit, and shifts us to a deeper experience of collectivity and connection. That experience of collective vibrational connection can change people on a neurological level and we may even begin to experience the power of that collective connection to effect change in the world. We may also find that we are more tuned in to our intuitive selves, receiving more information and able to speak our truth more powerfully.

One of the things we know is that in simply telling and listening to stories, there is a healing that happens. Deep and intense conflicts that can't be solved any other way can be helped through the act of compassionate listening. There can be no compassionate listening without an understanding of self-expression. That flow back and forth between the willingness to express myself to you and be seen by you and listen to who you are, shifts us. Ritual can create opportunities for this kind of storytelling and entering an exchange of communication with each other. Something happens in there that shifts us on a cellular level. It is an opportunity for practicing presence and that carries over to our day-to-day lives.

GRS: In some ways, those are the building blocks of ritual: self-expression, willingness to be present, compassionate listening to each other, entering a sacred space out of ordinary time, and opening to wonder.

SS: Yes! Ritual to me is about creating opportunities to connect with deeper parts of ourselves that live in both the eternal and mundane realms. We can bridge the two worlds through ritual, sound, color, any art really, because it speaks to the subverbal level of our being. We enter the mythological—what is beyond the five senses—and bring it into the world of five senses, allowing deeper meaning than we normally see. Often, this allows us to take on a larger perspective as well, and we revisit the possibility that there is a trajectory, a reason why I came to this planet, and things that I am here to do. Therefore, every part of life can be ritual. In Haiti, there is a phrase, "mountains beyond mountains" that I love. This can inspire us because there is always so much more than we can perceive. We must investigate those unknown places, all the scary and beautiful parts, and ritual can help us to do that.

Life is short and precious; it definitely has meaning. We don't have to let ourselves get too caught up in the distractions of entertainment and our lists of things to do. We lose that sense of purpose in our lives. We start to ask, "Wait, why am I here again, am I just taking up space or did I come to offer my gifts and receive the gifts of others?" We can have an ecstatic and inspired experience of life while we are in these miracle bodies. We don't have to give up our ability to connect with ourselves and with each other and ritual can offer us a moment to consciously create those opportunities.

GRS: What would you say is the difference between entertainment and ritual?

SS: I definitely came from a background as an entertainer. Entertainment has value—but it takes us out of our own lives. We watch reality television and get caught up in the drama of someone else's life. Ritual takes us into our own lives. What's behind the drama of my own life? I'm here to pursue my own purpose. What truly inspires is to have an even more embodied and yet mythical i.e., meaningful experience of your own life. What if everyone was living in their own movie; how would you live your life differently if film cameras were following you around?

GRS: What are the side effects of a world where people don't value ritual? What do you see as the major barriers to including these practices in the world we live in?

SS: The side effects are addiction, dysfunctional relationships, illness, disease, the ways we become "petty tyrants." In today's world, people don't feel empowered. There is a deification of gurus and performers, a pressure for them to give us art, to give our lives meaning. There is a deep shutdown of our connection with nature, the seasons, and any kind of change. There is a disconnection from the growing process, wisdom of age, only valuing certain standards of beauty. I'm shocked by the statistic that ninety-eight percent of people hate themselves because they don't fit a specific standard of attractiveness.

Some of the biggest barriers are the endless distractions of consumer culture, our critical minds shutting us down before we even get a chance to be creators, and also, ironically, the creation of "bad ritual." Right now, there is a lot of new age-ism that doesn't make any sense to the critical mind. Many of the rituals that are being created for the public are inaccessible. People see experimental things that are strange and say, "That doesn't work because I don't understand it." Ritual must include the neocortex; our thinking process is important. As we get better at this culturally, we can design ritual that speaks to both rational and mythological mind at same time. We begin to incorporate embodied practices that take us deeper into our bodies and include our minds and emotions. Ritual becomes a way that we can integrate all the parts of ourselves even more strongly.

GRS: What do you think would change in the world if ritual became integrated in our culture or available within our systems of medicine? For instance, what would be altered if medical practitioners included the suggestion to create ritual as an important factor in their recommendations for the treatment of illness?

SS: Some of most intense healing I have seen has included a mixture of the practical and the mythical. For example, loved ones going into surgery while their community is simultaneously doing ritual and prayer around it is a most powerful combination. If ritual as a tool was more integrated into our medical system, we might have an even deeper understanding of the mystery around illness and healing. We could acknowledge the possibility that illness is something for us to transmute or transform. We might call on the power of surrender and tap into our artistic selves for creative healing processes. It can be a deep teaching to explore the physical, mental, emotional, and spiritual habits and patterns that are not serving us and in fact are making us sick, and to take responsibility for finding a team of allies to assist in shifting those patterns. No one will do this for me, I have to go in and look at these patterns and honor how they have served me, and then begin to create ways of being that truly serve me at the deepest level. I have to also call on the divine invisible forces for support. It's tricky because the most difficult place is where superstition and science meet. We both want to believe in something that is bigger than us and we are afraid of it. Where we unwind superstition from fact, we find that there are things we think are indisputable "fact" in this moment but might not apply in five hundred years. Some things we think are a complete mystery right now might be a fact in five hundred years. Human beings are on a spectrum of evolution. It may be that we've gone so far in the direction of science and it's time to bring back practices that speak to the deeper parts of ourselves. We also know that our belief systems have a lot to do with our healing mechanisms. If we brought back belief systems that worked for us on a practical level, which connected us to nature and helped us to care for ourselves and for each other, those spiritual beliefs would shift things. But to me, any magical or spiritual practices must have practical applications! If these practices don't make me a better person enjoying my life or my community, they are not working.

Singing can be used as a metaphor for all this. For most people, singing is terrifying, but past that terror is a bliss that is undeniable and it changes people. In my ideal world, people would be a lot more self-expressive and would be using the sheer life force of expression for their own health and healing.

GRS: In your opinion, how would healers prescribe these practices of self-expression and ritual to create more holistic healing for people?

SS: Right now, doctors prescribe singing lessons for thyroid problems; through the vibration of the sound, the thyroid is stimulated. Singing is actually deeply physiologically healing, and hospitals are now experimenting with the creation of sound environments and specific sound practices for faster recovery from surgeries and other procedures. I think that rituals can be prescribed for people to help look at root causes; they can help move dis-ease and bring us into harmony with the self. I know that at the deepest scientific level of vibrational knowledge, the natural state of things is a harmony that is actually musically and mathematically sound.

Just like you do with Chinese medicine and acupuncture, we have to ask ourselves and our culture what is blocking the natural flow of vital life force? That is what ritual does; it brings us into natural relationship with the flow of vital life force. Any healer that would prescribe a practice that allows us to understand and speak our truth and that helps us to trust ourselves is contributing to our overall health. If we start creating ritual that takes us out of fear and into connection, deep healing occurs and begins to affect our whole life, and then spirit becomes part of everything. Our lives are no longer compartmentalized.

GRS: What is your offering to these interesting times in terms of your work? What does the world/what do humans need most right now in order to return to healthy culture?

SS: Part of healthy culture is the awareness that every action we take has an effect beyond our comprehension of that effect. We need to build an awareness of the times we are living in, using technology to connect as opposed to disconnect. Healthy culture would be a culture that is experiencing itself as having meaning and purpose. Part of my job is to continue to find my own creative expression, to help people find that self-expression for themselves, and to normalize healthy self-expression. Because I travel, I see that self-expression is a cross-cultural birthright, and I try to connect people with more indigenous rituals and make bridges between cultures.

We must keep creating ritual for these modern times. We don't always have to regurgitate the old rituals without meaning for us. Instead, we can ask what does it mean to create ritual now? What would it mean to connect people through ritual all over world, how can we move our collaboration forward, bring people together around common cause and ground? How do we understand each other through service, show up, look at root causes, and let go of old stories that wars are being fought over? Can we ask ourselves, "Now, what are we going to create?"

I see that the old forms and religions aren't working for people *and* that new age spouting doesn't work. What works is ritual that speaks to us, that is most intelligent, artistic, and real and still holds space for mystery. I think we can do it, but we must learn collaboration and listening and letting go of agendas. We can come to real practical understanding, not through just one spiritual tradition, but through what connects them all. There will have to be an evolution of the spirit to go along with this revolution of the spirit.

Perhaps the limited extent of the resources on the planet is a huge unifying factor. We now have capacity to relate to each other across the planet. Something else can be born, some way of being together spiritually that is both ecstatic and applicable to our everyday lives! People are waiting for permission and instruction. I want to give people permission to be self-expressive leaders for change. I would say to all healers, take a risk! Everyone is inherently creative, when people step into leadership or healing roles, start taking risks, then the magic will happen.

CHAPTER FIVE

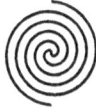

Creativity and Ecstasy: Twin Kisses of the Divine

Now you are no longer caught
in the obsession with darkness,
and a desire for higher love-making
sweeps you upward.
Distance does not make you falter,
now, arriving in magic, flying,
and, finally, insane for the light,
you are the butterfly and you are gone.
And so long as you haven't experienced
this: to die and so to grow,
you are only a troubled guest
on the dark earth.

– Goethe

We finish a hike on a trail in the Brisbane Ranges National Park in Victoria, Australia, and pile into the car to drive home. As we begin to pull away, three gray kangaroos hop out of the woods, crossing the road in front of us. They leap over a waist-high fence and propel themselves with legs and tails across the grassland away from us. White cockatoos screech in a nearby eucalyptus tree. We whisper to each other in soft tones that we have been blessed.

∞∞

My 39 year-old patient comes in to quit smoking cigarettes. We talk about the fact that many folks start out using substances as a way to experience joy, sensuality, and connection. She feels that there are very few places in her life where this is happening right now and we begin to figure out some ways to bring this into her life when she lets go of smoking. She decides on community dance classes, a new kind of chai tea, dried cherries, a break at work when she listens to her favorite music, a walk with her dog to the park in the evening, and a treat at the farmer's market each Saturday to mark the weeks that she does not smoke a cigarette.

Sacred Exploration:

Just as ritual can be a way to open the doorway to timeless space and vast imaginal potential, creativity and ecstasy connect with a presence larger than the human experience. Both of these concepts are often described as entering a flow of energy that leads to inspiration that flows through the artist or practitioner. Julia Cameron articulates this life force as "an underlying, in-dwelling creative force infusing all of life—including ourselves...we are ourselves, creations. And we, in turn are meant to continue creativity by being creative ourselves."[1] Ecstasy was the goal of the mystic in the past. Today it may live in the searches of both the spiritual and the agnostic human for healing. We are seeking joy and bliss, interruptions in the daily grind, opportunities to see beyond our own lives, to see into Spirit, to make art.

Neither ecstasy nor art is the same as escaping from our lives through addiction or shutting down our awareness to flee from situations that we find untenable. It is quite the opposite. Ideally, these pursuits feel like waking up, going beyond, expanding to embrace

82

something large and beautiful. Art can be grateful appreciation of the sensual detail in something small, like the exquisite detail in a seashell or a leaf. Ecstasy is deep and expansive, enormous and miniature. What brings you ridiculous amounts of pleasure? What would you do if you didn't have to earn a living? The answers to these questions are often your treasure, your secret creative revolutionary soul.

Creativity is another name for grace, another name for homo sapiens. All the arts have been proven for thousands of years to heal body, mind and spirit. Our creative expression is part of our human genius. We can make and build and move and manifest beauty or powerful forms of resistance with art. And it is through art, that humans have sought ecstasy.

Creativity and ecstasy are streams of the same river. Humans will always seek ecstatic experiences that bring us to the mystical place of merging our edges into all that is. Cross-cultural anthropological studies have shown that we take drugs, meditate, practice yoga, ingest psychedelic herbs and plants, dance, chant, fast, pray, breathe, and really anything else we can think of to feel ourselves part of something bigger. Ecstasy helps to dissolve the limited ego view of the self and fill with a wider expression of life, touching the divine, building a communion with Spirit that often defies language. So does art.

Ecstasy is too big to fit inside one religion. The Jewish faith has Qabalah, Christianity has Gnosticism, and the Muslims have Sufism. Many have tried to eradicate it from the repertoire of their particular tradition over the years by calling people crazy or heretic. There are religions that reserve the ecstatic experience for trained priests or professionals or guard the practices as secret.

These days, the pathways to creative arts and ecstasy are wide open to the masses. Art lessons and guides to ecstatic practices are available through teachers, books, music, the internet and YouTube. There has never been a time on earth when these experiences have been so accessible to so many. Why are they so desirable? What is it about creativity and ecstasy that keeps us coming back for more?

Ecstasy gives us a feeling of unity. The Sufi tradition would say that our romantic relationships mimic the bliss we feel when we connect with Spirit. These experiences obliterate our loneliness for a while and bring us back into communion. It is difficult to find words to describe this; it is greater, larger, wiser, and more joyful than our everyday experience.

Many of us only associate ecstasy with sex and romance. These are certainly ways to ecstasy but they are not very reliable over the long haul. Most of the time, the idealistic projections that we have about a new lover eventually give way to a more realistic picture of who that person is. If we are dependent on romance to take us to ecstasy, we can end up very dissatisfied in our relationships. It is too high an expectation of anyone to "make us feel" ecstatic all the time! If we can create our own doorways to ecstasy and creativity, we can relax and feel confident that we will have another blissful visit again soon.

Jalaja Bonheim, therapist and author, discusses ecstasy as a human birthright and argues that most problems with substances or other addictions are a botched search for ecstatic experience.[2] It is not an accident that many addictive substances produce changes in our neurochemistry. It is possible that the substances that we imbibe, inhale, or consume take the place of communion with a larger source. Did the decrease in opportunities for ecstasy drive us to change our neurochemistry through other means? If this joy and passion are meant to be ours, what has happened to take us so far away from the arts that lead to ecstasy?

What kind of art makes people feel joyful? Author and activist Barbara Ehrenreich explores this question from the perspective of joyful experiences that happen in a community setting. Many cultures throughout the world had dancing, singing, and festivals as part of their regular lives. There have been pathways through religion or ceremony, celebrations or sporting events to create camaraderie, good will, and fun. For many people cross-culturally and throughout time, work is physically difficult and life carries many threats of violence or health scares on a day-to-day basis. Ehrenreich reminds us that "to extract pleasure from lives of grinding hardship and oppression is a considerable accomplishment; to achieve ecstasy is a kind of triumph."[3] She outlines the routes that organized religion has taken to outlaw these activities and postulates that this is an attempt to control joy. She further theorizes that people who have access to joy, ecstasy, and celebration are difficult to control by any external authority.[4]

Both art and ecstasy have an unfortunate association with shame for many people. There are many voices in the world telling us that we should not feel bliss, we don't deserve to make art, because we have too many obligations. The truth is that ecstasy is a need that will eventually find a way to be met. When we don't make space for creativity and ecstasy in our lives, we make ourselves vulnerable to seeking it in the shadows, in experiences that we would not consciously choose. It is an all too familiar story when people put themselves in situations that are completely opposite to their life circumstances or create situations that cause other people pain in order to find a peak experience and then feel ashamed of doing so. Illicit love affairs, anonymous sexual encounters, secret addictions are all ways that we beg for ecstasy. We don't have to be beggars in our own lives. If we can learn to hear our own cries for our creative souls a little sooner, we can answer the call in ways that are healthier. I believe it is fully possible to attend to our responsibilities and to cultivate regular excursions to visit creative arts and ecstatic bliss.

Ecstasy holds within it the understanding or belief that we are not alone. It may even be that we need to believe that we are not the highest rung on the evolutionary ladder or that our daily lives are not the only way we can live. Ecstatic experience may bring us closer to this understanding than any other.

Ecstasy is sometimes the pinnacle of human experience and sometimes the abyss. We tend to seek the pinnacle and shun the abyss but life can have other plans for us. Even in our grief sometimes, we can find a larger ecstatic truth. If we are able to stay in touch with our feelings, even when it means experiencing discomfort, we seem to move through emotions more quickly and with grace. Creative expression of all kinds helps us do this. Shutting down emotions can seem like a short-term solution to avoid pain but it rarely ends in long-term health.

Physical movement, especially the art of dance, can help us process very large emotions and get to the other side of them. I often recommend going dancing after a breakup or loss and really letting your body express itself. Giving our body the language of dance when we are experiencing negative emotions can help us access a place that is ecstatic, connecting with something bigger than our pain.

Singing is another pathway to ecstasy. When we sing, we open ourselves in ways that tear down our normal defenses and steers us toward health, as Suzanne Sterling discusses in Chapter 3. Singing can change our mood and shift our emotions. Sound can also help us express things when words fail us. I have used singing, chanting, and toning in sessions to help patients break through very stuck places and release stagnant emotions. During the early days of my divorce, I sang (and sometimes yelled and wept) every day. Making the sound of grief gave it a voice and a way to move through my body.

Rhythm helps to rewire the emotional systems. Our bodies sometimes move to a drumbeat without thinking about it. Drums have been used by many cultures to induce trance states and rhythm is often a container for ecstatic dancing or vocalization. Listening to drums changes our neurological systems whether we like it or not.

Compassion is a quality that is often revered in the world's mystery traditions. It is basically empathy on a deep level for another being, the understanding or identifying with another's suffering. To be alive is to experience pain and joy alike. We all have this capacity. We can support each other best when we open to compassion for each other's experiences. This, too, is a part of creativity and ecstasy.

Joanna Macy takes an ecstatic approach in her "work that reconnects" (Chapter 2). Instead of ignoring or closing off the difficult truths about the environment and other global problems, she dives right into them.[5] As we learn from this work, opening ourselves can bring us together with other humans experiencing the same emotions that we are. The only way out of grief and pain may be through it. If we go together, we support and advise each other. From there, we are always able to be more creative about where to go next.

It is not a coincidence that many of the practices that create ecstasy have been commandeered in our culture by industry. We get social training very early in industrialized culture about who should dance, sing, drum or draw and who should not. We must heal this damage around creativity in order to find the beauty of communion with Spirit. There is much to do in reclaiming our imaginative bodies and our voices for the work of ecstasy. If we can let go of the harmful story that only those with clear talents that show up immediately should ever create any kind of art, we may discover that we have the seeds of talents that no one has yet seen. If you were ever a magical child who never received the support to become yourself, see yourself now. You are the most sacred darling and your need to play and create is one of the most divine things about you. Rest assured, you are not entitled to be the best at everything but you have the absolute right to take a holy risk and begin. It is never too late to begin doing something that you have always wanted to try. It is not bad to do it awkwardly, to fall on your face and giggle. Just begin.

Even without a clear and recognized skill for a specific art, we can practice all the methods of creativity available to us and find them meaningful or fun.

T. Thorn Coyle, author, activist, and internationally respected teacher of esoteric spiritual arts, speaks about where ecstasy converges with her work, in conversation about our collective health. "Choosing to open up space for the sacred is one of the most healing things we can do for ourselves and for all our relationships.

In a world that can feel so broken by war, environmental devastation, and personal or community crisis, anything that helps us to reintegrate with a larger whole can lead to healing. If we are all part of the unfolding divine process of the cosmos, along with the trees, animals, water, stars, and beings seen and unseen, then there is simply nothing to transcend. We are light in extension and we are the fertile darkness from which all things are born. There is uniqueness and a sameness that simultaneously dance. We are cells in the body of All That Is."

What if it is part of our human birthright to create art, sing, dance, and find ecstasy no matter what is happening in our lives, in the world? Despite the pain, the wars, the crises that continue to mark human lives all over the planet, still we rise, still we sing, still we create music and ritual as if we must. Our hearts might be broken open and still we find joy in unlikely places. There is rarely a moment when we are not in search of comfort, strength, freedom, or belonging. Our seeking of these things, our raw need for them can open us to the possibility of feeling them, even if just in moments of ecstasy.

Glimpses of a larger pattern can provide sustenance and motivation. What really matters? Creativity can help us to remember and redefine our answers or at least help us continue to pray for revelation. Western culture defines it as weakness to open the heart or show any kind of vulnerability. Ecstasy and art will allow us more ways to participate in life's dance of loving and letting go.

Revolutionary Healing Dares:

I dare you to begin practicing an art that you always wanted to try but didn't think you would be any good at it. I dare you to make terrible art that will make you laugh and your inner censor scream. I dare you to sing and dance and let yourself take up space in the world and even in your own body. I dare you to find a regular way to lose your intellectual monkey mind and join something bigger and brighter than you can imagine. I dare you to remind someone else of this truth as well, to open someone else's eyes to their connection with All That Is.

I dare you to express this need for ecstasy and creativity online and in person, to stand for the right brain's joyful niche to merge and blend with all that is, in compassionate company. I dare you to talk about what is terrifying you about the world right now and ask people to hold space for you. I dare you to offer to hold space for other people to express their terrors. I dare you to find a community that is willing to celebrate emotions of grief, joy, fear, comfort, anger; let every single human emotion find a home. I dare you to be part of that.

Spiritual Inventory:
Exercises for Ecstasy

1. **Joy explorer:** For the next three months, give yourself permission to try something once a week that might bring you joy. These can be activities or practices that you already know are pleasurable for you *or* things that you have never tried before. If you are drawing a blank thinking about them, ask yourself: What did I once love to do and now it's too silly or too expensive or too much trouble? What would I try if I knew I would be good at it right away? What would I experiment with if I knew it could not fail and no one would laugh?

2. **Time travel letters:** Write a letter to yourself from five years in the future. Pretend that you are five years older giving advice to yourself in the present time. Tell yourself exactly what to do to increase happiness and opportunities for ecstatic connection. If you are having trouble conceiving of this, let yourself remember where you were in your life five years ago. Start with a letter to yourself back then to console or encourage yourself in your

struggles during that period of your life. Especially take note of the problems that you had then that have since been solved and the ideas or dreams that you have been able to manifest.

3. **Connection:** Ecstasy is often about a feeling of connection to something larger and beautiful. Where do you feel that now or where do you suspect that you might feel that in the future? What do you personally believe about God, Goddess or Spirit or Creative Intelligence? Are there memories or experiences in your life where you felt that was real?

4. **Slow down:** Sit down with your calendar again. Pick a time once per week to turn off screens, phones, computers, and anything you feel is a distraction or a motivation to move very fast. Stay in this space for at least an hour and either do nothing or do something that does not require a high degree of technology to perform.

5. **Go outside:** In most places we can dress for the weather and spend a little time outside several times a week. What is the difference between the air outside and inside? What do your senses tell you about what is going on outside? Where is your favorite place to be outside that is possible to get to within twenty minutes? Is there any errand or activity in your life to which you can walk or ride? What do you see or hear in different seasons?

Living Inspiration: Jalaja Bonheim

I met with Jalaja Bonheim to discuss the importance of creative ecstasy and her recent book, *Evolving Toward Peace*. Jalaja is an author, counselor, and international leader of workshops. She is the founder of Circlework, a process that she has taken into schools and other venues all over the world to reclaim the sacred and introduce peaceful alternatives to our culture.

GRS: Where do you personally see a hunger for the sacred the most?

JB: I see it in every aspect of life. Actually, there is nowhere that I *don't* see it. We are in such a crisis. Humans are an endangered species, and this awareness is intensifying our yearning for a deeper connection to spirit and to ourselves. I see a growing awareness that the way we've been living is no longer working. More and more people understand that we have lost our way. It's a painful awareness, but it's also acting as an incentive for awakening and change.

The main practice that I teach is Circlework, a method that uses circle gatherings to heal individuals and communities. The circle is an ancient and universal format for community gatherings; all traditional peoples gathered in circles to strengthen their community, but also to commune with spirit. I don't usually describe it as an ecstatic practice, but it most definitely is. When people in a circle really connect with each other and with spirit, it's totally ecstatic.

These days, many groups meet in circles, but in general, there's a lack of skill. The circle is a powerful tool, but people haven't learned how to effectively use it. So that is what I teach. Many participants in my circles are healers, educators, and activists who want to bring the gifts of the circle to their communities. But there are also business people, ministers, and rabbis.

One of the beauties of the circle is that you don't have to name the spiritual component of what is happening. And by not naming it, you can bypass people's defenses. For example, I have a client who is a corporate executive and who leads circles in corporations. She's definitely helping people connect with their spirituality, but she doesn't call it that.

Traditional religion used to be responsible for helping people commune with spirit and to experience the ecstasy of that connection. But today, most people are no longer getting that from religion. They aren't finding the nourishment their hearts and souls crave.

Circlework is not a substitute for religion. Rather, it's a non-religious spiritual practice that allows people of every religion and culture to come together in unity and receive the deep nourishment, healing, and connection they hunger for. It provides a container that is safe and respectful and, at the same time, profoundly sacred.

In my circles, there's a strong emphasis on receptivity and gentleness. For many people, this is a very new experience and very different than what the dominant culture propagates. There is no pressure to do anything. But when people witness someone else having an emotional or ecstatic opening, it often gives them the courage to allow their own authentic self-expression.

We're all afraid of being judged, so we need safe, protected spaces to explore new ways of being and relating. I hope that we find a way to loosen our powerful attachments to certain beliefs. We can have beliefs, and that's fine, but we can no longer afford to base our sense of identity on them.

It's ironic that religion tends to encourage belief addiction, even though it's actually an obstacle to true spirituality. The sacred is after all not a mental experience. Ecstasy doesn't happen through the mind. If you've been taught it's wrong to question your beliefs or let them go, you've got a major barrier to ecstatic connection.

Another huge barrier is patriarchy. I'm not talking just about the oppression of women. Patriarchy has also led to the rejection of everything our culture labels feminine, including gentleness, beauty, grace, nature, and the body. All religions that have incorporated patriarchal beliefs, such as Hinduism, Buddhism, Christianity, and Islam, have also incorporated the belief that spirit is separate from matter and that we need to transcend the body. Of course this makes it difficult for us to connect with our body's innate capacity for ecstasy.

In our culture, all the symptoms of the heart's opening, such as vulnerability, sensitivity, and softness, are associated with the feminine. As a result, they've been burdened with shame. This is especially true for men, but to some extent, women, too, suffer from what I call "heartshame." Heartshame is one of the main weapons patriarchy uses to scare us away from embracing our feminine side. Heartshame is a major obstacle to ecstasy, because to open to ecstasy, we have to let go of control. And what patriarchy teaches us is that we're supposed to be in control at all times.

GRS: What do you think would change in the world if creative or ecstatic practices became integrated in our culture or available within our systems of medicine?

JB: That would be so wonderful! It would lead to an entirely different vision of what it means to be human. I think the whole medical system would have to change dramatically. Of course it would also radically change the nature of medical training. Right now Western medicine approaches the body exclusively as a physical object. If these practices went mainstream, physicians would have to approach their patients as emotional and spiritual beings as well.

I would love to see circles available everywhere, including hospitals. Right now, nurses are always caring for others, but they have no place where *they* can receive healing and nurturance. For patients, it would be equally valuable. Research shows that cancer patients who have a strong support circle live longer. If every hospital had a trained circle facilitator who could offer a truly healing environment for both the patients and the staff, it would make an enormous difference.

GRS: What would be altered if medical practitioners included the development of an ecstatic practice as an important factor in their recommendations for the treatment of illness?

JB: Well, we need to keep in mind that words are tricky. The very word *ecstasy* can trigger fear and resistance. I think it's important that practitioners try to use words their patients are comfortable with. We need to meet people where they are. *Ecstasy* is a word that many people find challenging. But there are questions we can ask without using that word. Where does someone find an opening to connect with spirit or with a sense of the sacred? For one person it might be gardening. For another, it might be music or being with animals. It takes skill to talk about these things with patients. You want to talk in ways that don't turn them off or scare them.

Of course, for medical practitioners to recommend ecstatic practices, they themselves would have to have experience with such practices. It would also require a lot of personal growth on their part. In their training, far more attention would need to be given to the cultivation of compassion and empathy. Right now fear tends to keep physicians separate from patients. They're afraid of connecting with the patient's suffering and vulnerability. In particular, I find the current emphasis on keeping people alive at any cost horrible and perverse. It's a symptom of our profound distrust of nature and of our body's innate wisdom.

GRS: We have discussed that creative work often leads to ecstasy. Do you have other examples of words or questions that healers could use to help the patient get to an ecstatic practice?

JB: We might ask: What gives you a sense of well-being? What makes you happy? If you were to make happiness the first priority in your life, what would change? If you were to make pleasure a primary priority, what would change? We want to create a space where people can be authentic and honest and won't feel judged. Everyone carries within themselves the knowledge of what they need. So instead of telling them what to do, can we help them connect to that inner source? If we can create a space for folks to articulate what they need and what makes them happy, that is a great first step.

Sometimes I invite people to imagine who they'll be when they are very old and close to dying. What would that person say to them now? Often this leads to a tremendous outpouring of wisdom. Usually, that voice tells them to stop worrying and spend more time doing what they love.

GRS: What is your offering to these interesting times in terms of your work?

JB: My two greatest passions are peace and the sacred feminine. I have a strong commitment to empowering the feminine in our world. Working with women in the Middle East and with women from Afghanistan has been eye-opening because it has really showed me how immense the degree of oppression is and how far we still have to go. In the US, women have a great deal of freedom and equality, but this is not the case in a huge portion of the world.

I am committed to creating sisterhood between women around the world. Women need to support each other, because until women are respected and free, we won't have a healthy world. I would go so far as to say that the whole imbalance of our culture can be traced back to the loss of balance between the masculine and the feminine. Sexuality is after all one of the most important ecstatic practices. But for sexuality to serve as a gateway to ecstasy, people need to be true partners. In a world where all genders are at odds with each other, the barriers to intimacy and ecstasy are enormous.

GRS: How would you help someone cultivate an ecstatic practice?

JB: I would ask that person what they love. If they said, "I love dancing," I would invite them to make dancing a high priority in their lives. What you love is your access to ecstasy. No one can tell you how to find it. But others can help you discover where your access lives. Ecstasy is not something we can control. We should never think, "If I do this, I can have ecstasy." It's a gift of grace. We can create environments or circumstances under which ecstasy is more likely to arise, but then we must surrender. We can't *make* it happen or force it to come when we call. This is an important component in the problem of addiction. We think we have found something we can depend on to lead us into ecstasy, so we keep coming back to it. But it doesn't work that way. We can't control the creative or the divine. We can only open to it.

GRS: What does the world/what do humans need most right now in order to return to healthy culture?

JB: On a very practical note, I think we need to slow down. We are all moving too fast and doing too much. We live far too much in our heads. We need to stop, step out of our minds and into nature, into our bodies so we can listen to the profound source of wisdom that lies within us.

These experiences give us the support and encouragement we need to take this more authentic way of being out into our lives and our relationships.

I just completed a new book called *Evolving Toward Peace: Awakening the Global Heart.* In it, I look at the way that our collective consciousness is changing and *must* change if our species is to survive. I don't believe we change in isolation. Rather, we change in connection with one another. And today, many people long to experience a sense of spiritual presence, not just alone in nature, or in prayer and meditation, but also in their relationships. They're looking for a sense of sacred presence that can infuse their relationships with the fragrance of ecstasy, and that can connect them with a true spiritual community. In our times, the vast majority of people don't have anything close.

GRS: What does ecstasy mean to you? How did ecstatic practices come to be a vital part of your life and work? Why is it of value to you?

JB: I like that Greek word *ecstasis*, which means, "to stand outside of." In ecstasy, we step beyond our ego. The ego dissolves, at least temporarily. That's tremendously liberating, especially for us, who live in such an ego-based culture. We yearn to shed the weight of the ego and become one with something greater than our small ego-self. We long for the experience of oneness, whether it's with spirit, with a person or an animal, even a tree or a piece of music.

For me, dancing is an important path to ecstasy. In *Aphrodite's Daughters*, I wrote about my experience of studying Indian temple dance. In my research into the practices of the Indian temple dancers, I found that they were not just dancers but priestesses. Like the witches of medieval times, they were healers and midwives; they accompanied the dying, and they lived and worked in community.

I came to the US in 1982. At that time, I began to lead circles, and I've been doing so ever since. My circles never included Indian dance. And yet, we too enter into sacred space; the circle becomes our temple. So you might say that the circles I lead are modern day expressions of what the Indian priestesses used to do in ancient times.

I think we all long to step outside the confines of daily life and merge with something greater. We need to find ways of coming together in community to acknowledge, address, and honor that hunger. All indigenous communities had celebrations, rituals, ways that allowed the entire community to tap into that source of ecstasy. We've lost the traditional ways. So now, we have to discover our own.

GRS: Why is ecstatic connection or practice important to our collective health?

JB: Ecstasy is as important to our well-being as food, drink, and shelter. We can go without it for a while, but if this need isn't addressed, we'll turn to unhealthy ways to fulfill it.

Personally, I think that in our society, most people are suffering from a kind of spiritual starvation. Without connection to spirit, life feels barren and dry. There are many consequences: high rates of suicide—especially among youth—depression, drug use, violence.

In *The Hunger for Ecstasy*, I wrote about addiction, and how many forms of addiction are expressions of a yearning for ecstasy that isn't being addressed. The result is that we look to substitutes like alcohol, drugs, and shopping. How come so many people are attracted to a recreational drug like ecstasy? Waging a war on drugs is not the answer. We need to realize that people are trying to satisfy a very real and irrepressible need.

I believe our failure to provide socially accepted ways to experience ecstasy also fuels our attraction to violence. Growing up in Germany after World War II, I remember listening to the men talk about their war memories. I came to understand that for many, those direct encounters with danger, pain, and death had transported them to an edge where pain can flip over into ecstasy. Even though their experiences had been horrific, they felt a kind of nostalgia because they no longer had a way of accessing that edge.

To me, the essence of spirituality is the experience of oneness with the world, which is inherently ecstatic. If such experiences were commonplace, I don't see how there could be war. Once you realize in a visceral, embodied way that we are one, you can no longer harm others without feeling that you are harming yourself.

GRS: What do you see as the major barriers to including ecstatic practices in the world we live in?

JB: One of the major barriers, which I address in *Evolving Toward Peace*, is something I call "belief addiction." For thousands of years, we were taught to define who we were based on the beliefs we held—typically the beliefs of our tribe. The fact that we held those beliefs identified us as a member of the tribe. It bonded us to our people and formed the basis of our identity. But beliefs are inherently divisive. They bond us with our tribe, but they also separate us from everyone else.

Today, we need to embrace our oneness as a global community otherwise we will have no future. So this habit of basing our identity on specific beliefs has now become unsustainable.

Right now, we're destroying nature, the very basis of our survival. To come back into harmony with the world in which we live, we need to realign ourselves with the rhythms of nature, which are much slower than the rhythms of industrial culture. We are addicted to speed as a way of running from ourselves. One of the first things we do in my retreats is slow down and come home to ourselves. Until we are one with ourselves, how can we do anything worthwhile?

CHAPTER SIX

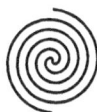

Soul Restoration:
The Call Our Souls Must Answer

Hard to Forget
I was waiting for the
longest time, she said.
I thought you forgot.
It is hard to forget, I
said, when there is
such an empty space
when you are gone.

— BRIAN ANDREAS

*A*t age nineteen, I am diagnosed with cervical cancer and follow
my doctor's suggestions to have surgery to remove it. Ever since, I
have had painful menstrual cramps that do not respond to pain-
killers. A number of medical doctors have not been able to give any
further direction other than a diagnosis of endometriosis and the suggestion of more surgery that may or may not help. I begin to pursue some
alternative healing for my reproductive health problems. I want to fully
heal myself and prevent future occurrences. I am in Santa Fe, sitting in

a counseling session with a friend of a friend who is a counselor and also does shamanic work. I don't know exactly what shamanic work means at first, so she explains what soul retrieval is. I identify with many of the symptoms she describes and realize that I have indeed felt numb and disconnected from my body since the surgery. She tells me that it is possible that a piece of myself was left behind during that event and that it may be time for that part to come home to join the rest of me. I feel hot tears on my cheeks when she says this, though I don't understand why.

∞

My 41 year-old patient has experienced a miscarriage and comes to be treated for abdominal pain and depression. She has a difficult time making eye contact with me and says she has not been able to leave the house for two weeks. When she is lying on the table, I ask her to let go of any parts of her body that she is still holding up, to pretend she can sink two more inches into the table. We do a meditation where she envisions her attention as a web of energetic strands. With her breath, she begins calling back the strands of energy and attention and imagines returning them to her body. She chooses to gather them in her belly. After a few minutes, she sighs audibly and opens her eyes and looks directly at me. "Wow, I was very far away before I did that."

Sacred Exploration:

The reality of modern living is that we do not spend all of our time in embodied connection with land, creating rituals that lead us to blissful and ecstatic states. Life happens and some life experiences can be excruciating. We survive the encounters themselves and make progress, but afterward, it may seem as if something has vanished. We may not be able to put words to what has disappeared. We hear stories from friends, family, patients, and clients about the ways that life situations become worse in slow gradations over time. The circumstances are almost but not quite intolerable and yet, there is no end in sight, no clear escape route. We can't be certain that it is an emergency so we don't ask for help.

In Siberian lore, Chinese medicine, Celtic spirituality, and South American tribal religions, a common cross-cultural belief is that when a traumatic event is experienced, the soul splits apart and pieces of it disappear. Whether this soul loss is viewed as a physical malady or a metaphor, this concept is too widespread over many different continents to be a coincidence. This archetype of a lost soul part returning home to join the whole must have rang true for many humans.

In ancient China, the Shen were considered to be helping spirits that were developed by a person following the Tao or "the way." One of my teachers of acupuncture and alchemy, Lorie Dechar, told us a myth from Taoist philosopher, Chuang Tzu, about the Shen taking the form of golden birds that nested in the calm center of a person's heart. During trauma or shock, the birds might take flight because the heart became so agitated and stormy that there was no place for them to rest.[1] In the times before the diagnosis of shock, Chinese healers and shamans would encourage people to calm their centers and make a space for the Shen to come home and rest. Whenever I share this story about the Shen birds flying away with my acupuncture patients or my students, there is a look that flashes across their faces, as if they are recognizing an old friend. We all want those birds to come home.

In ancient Celtic medical practices, there was also a treatment called soul restoration for calling the soul back to the body. Healers would suggest practices of realignment that their patients would perform daily leading up to the soul restoration ritual. There was an emphasis on attuning three states of being, perhaps not dissimilar to our concepts of body, mind, and spirit. Author and Celtic scholar, Caitlin Matthews, describes the catalyst for this soul restoration process: "The trinity of the soul, heart, and mind are strong in harmony, yet they can be shattered if they are not in union. Doubt, distrust, and neglected observances are the pathways to madness, heartsickness, and soul fragmentation."[2] Healers would also pray for grace on the other's behalf because it was a widespread belief that people could not bring back their own souls by themselves, once pieces had departed. Music was a vital part of this soul restoration; healers would use music as a template to reconstruct the soul parts into a whole. There may have been potential for other community members to be involved in this healing process.[3]

There are no distinct ways to measure the effectiveness of this kind of working, whether it was a ritual or a procedure. We don't know how long it took, how satisfied people were afterward. It is known however that this did not happen once with one person but repeatedly with thousands of people all over the world who sought healing because they felt disconnected from their lives. Clearly, someone experienced some relief after a soul restoration!

Many of my patients who have been in car accidents often describe a condition similar to soul loss. They feel "fuzzy," as if they are not quite all there. Even without severe injuries, people frequently express that they are frightened to get back in the car or to drive on the same road where they experienced the crash. Many tell me they have had difficulty sleeping or they have nightmares where they relive the accident. In other times and cultures, it is possible that this would have been treated with some kind of soul recovery.

Disassociation or even shock are immediate responses after traumatic events that function to protect the body, mind, and spirit. People report physical numbness, stray thoughts that do not fit the circumstances, sensations of being far away, changes in vision, drops in body temperature, and confusion. Ideally, with care and over time, this situation shifts and the brain can begin to process the trauma and integrate the new circumstances. What do we do as healers when this does not happen?

Sometimes the symptoms of disassociation are not apparent even to the person who is experiencing them. In my own life situation at nineteen, I had not really tracked my own divorce from my body after my surgery; I would have told anyone who asked that I was doing fine and had completely recovered from the surgery. However, if someone asked further questions, they would have discovered that my interest in sex had decreased, I wasn't writing down the dates of my menstrual periods, I was taking a great deal of ibuprofen every month to dull my brutal cramps, my alcohol use had increased. I was often close to tears for no particular reason, and I didn't have much hope of anything changing. I had decided that I would tough it out until perhaps I needed more surgery. I never would have considered soul retrieval as one of the potential treatments; my problems were purely physical! And yet, my response to the surgery permeated all parts of my life.

Although treatment for trauma is an ancient discipline, treatment for post-traumatic stress syndrome has improved dramatically since contemporary research began in the 1960s with Vietnam War veterans. People who are diagnosed with PTSD now have a variety of options, including medication, therapy, and bodywork. Many of the latest treatments focus on releasing somatic memories that are stored in the body's muscle tissues. Francine Shapiro, the pioneer of EMDR (eye movement desensitization and reprocessing), developed a remarkable system to surpass the conscious mind and access old trauma stored in a deeper part of the brain. Trauma survivors experience EMDR as helping them to rewire their bodies and reduce their reactions to stress.

EMDR has proven effective for war veterans and survivors of sexual assault and it has also been translated for use with folks whose trauma might not be of that nature. The lens of trauma can be used to illustrate a wide variety of experiences. Healers are finding more and more, with the addition of stress, our bodies are sometimes reacting to regular life events as if they were traumatic. As discussed in our work with Embodiment, many of us have adrenaline in our systems on a daily basis and not usually because we are engaged in fighting or fleeing from predators or adversaries. This certainly has an urgent effect on the kinds of decisions we are making.

The symptoms of PTSD are becoming more common or more recognized all over the world, even in the absence of violent trauma: insomnia, depression, anxiety, hypervigilance, suspicion, easy startle response. What conclusion can global revolutionary healers draw from this? What is needed for people to feel safe in the world, fully present in their bodies? How can the healing practice of soul restoration inspire and inform the healing we use today to call home the parts of the soul that feel lost?

Somatic Experiencing (SE) and the work of Peter Levine is one way to embody this process. In his book, *In An Unspoken Voice*, Levine describes trauma as happening when the body's natural "discharges are inhibited, resisted, prevented from completion, our natural rebounding abilities get stuck." He advocates strongly for allowing the nervous system to follow its natural tendency to release trauma through preconditioned responses to stimuli. He states that when this cannot happen, people are more likely to suffer from PTSD afterward. "Trauma occurs when we are intensely frightened and are either physically restrained or perceive that we are trapped...If stuck in trauma, we can't discover the transitory nature of despair, terror, rage, and helplessness and that the body is designed to cycle in and out of these extremes."[4]

Levine goes on to describe a healthy sympathetic nervous system as utilizing options that he refers to as the A and four F's. First, a potential threat is perceived. The body almost always goes into "Arrest (increased vigilance and scanning), Flight (try first to escape), Fight (if the animal or person is prevented from escaping), Freeze (fright—scared stiff), Fold (collapse into helplessness).[5]

Practitioners of Somatic Experiencing are trained to help people reenter the places in their nervous systems that may be stuck in a previous traumatic situation. This can show up in body pain or unexplained symptoms that Western medicine practitioners cannot explain with MRIs, lab tests, or X-rays. Such symptoms may be reduced to 'hypochondriac or psychosomatic' pain and the patient may not receive the care needed to transform the root of the problem. PTSD complaints can also be a result of a nervous system that has not completed its release of stress/fear from a traumatic event.

In shamanic cultures (particularly the Tungus people of Siberia), practitioners journey to another realm to call back the soul part for the individual after a split. In this culture, we help our patients and clients reset their nervous systems through various techniques like body-based therapy, massage, acupuncture, Somatic Experiencing, EMDR, Feldenkrais, hypnosis, Focusing, and other methods of tuning into the body in order to transform the experience of trauma and restore a sense of wholeness.

On a more immediate scale, we can encourage people to call back their scattered attention from all the stimulating distractions in the world, all the lists of things to do and all the future worries. Before I start many acupuncture sessions, I ask my patients to do some breathing and imagine their attention as strands of energy "stuck" to people, places, and problems. Once they indicate that they can visualize this, I ask them to use their breath to release the hold of their attention strands on all these things and pull them back in, returning their attention to their own bodies. I ask that they find a place on their body to gather their attention, and use language like, "All pieces of my attention, focus, and energy come home to this body." People often visibly relax, and their exhalations get deeper and longer. They report feeling more present, focused, and in their bodies.

Perhaps it is similar to the feeling of the Shen spirits finding a space to return in their centers.

Soul loss may also be a great frame for the suffering in our culture. Perhaps one explanation from some of the painful experiences of war and destruction in our culture is that we are suffering from collective soul loss, separation from what is of importance. Many beautiful things about human culture have been dissected in a long series of traumatic events or just through forgetting. Our collective Shen spirits may have flown the coop, leaving us empty hearted and a little lost.

Every human life contains pain, because we are finite and so much of what we love is temporary. However, we have the capacity to heal from trauma, to allow our nervous systems to restore themselves, and to feel whole and healthy again. If we find inspiration in the concept of soul restoration, we can remind ourselves that everything lost can be found again, that we can call ourselves and each other back from places that seem scary or dreadful.

If soul recovery is effective for individuals, how might it work for our culture? There are pieces of our humanity that we can name and invite back in, especially the things that bring us joy, connection, honor, community, and deeper relationship with the world around us. We are already doing this. We can increase or renew our efforts.

Revolutionary Healing Dares:

I dare you to ask yourself where you feel numb and disconnected from yourself and use journaling or meditation to notice when it started and what pieces of you are asking to return home. I dare you to take some time in your day to invite your attention and energy back from all the situations that have called it away and encourage those around you to do the same. I dare you to do this publicly, in meetings, sessions, performances. I dare you to seek healing for your nervous system and find sustainable ways to renew your energy after stressful periods of time. I dare you to consider the possibility for yourself and for those you touch that trauma is finite and that there is always a chance at healing, redemption, support, hope, wholeness. I dare you to live as if personal and collective trauma can be healed.

Spiritual Inventory:
Exercises for Soul Restoration

1. **Soul retrieval meditation:** Sit or lie down in a comfortable position and close your eyes. You can record this meditation yourself, have someone else read it to you, or read it through 2-3 times and trust you will remember what is important.

   Notice the weight of your body against the surface you are touching. Feel the places where your body meets what is holding you up. Remind yourself that you don't have to hold yourself up right now; let any parts of your body that you are still holding up relax fully. You may find that you sink in a few inches as you stop holding up your own body weight. Remind yourself that there is nothing that you need to take care of right now in this moment. Allow yourself to turn around to face inside yourself and open your inner eyes. Begin to imagine your energy as strands of a web that extends from you into all the parts of your life. Everything that you notice or give attention to gets at least one strand of your attention.

   When you can see that web with you as its center, you can start to use your breath to unstick, untie, or unfasten those strands of your energy and attention from all the places, people, situations, and tasks to which they are attached. One by one, the strands begin to come home to you. Your breath is the invitation for your energy to come home to you, strand by strand. Just for now, all your attention returns. If you want, you can choose a place on your body to gather up your energy, restoring it to you. Breathe in and let it come home and gather it up for your own work, for your own healing. You can always extend it outward again, but right now, this is your focus, your energy, your attention.

2. **Forgiveness lists:** If you are having a hard time knowing where parts of yourself might be stuck, you can make a list of the more challenging events of your life. Begin as young as you remember and move through what you imagine to be the places where you experienced a hard time. If you notice an emotional charge or some bodily discomfort around a specific event, make a note of it. Another list that can elucidate these spaces where there is

emotional work to be done is a list of people who have hurt us and a list of those to whom we may have caused harm, whether accidentally or purposefully. It is easy to notice with this list where we may still have some buried feelings or where we might have some more expression to do. It often happens that our mind feels fine about the outcome of a situation while our body is still holding onto some part of it. Letting go of shame and blame is often key to "emptying" the emotional space. Are there any reparations or expressions of regret that need to be made to yourself or another person?

3. **Come home letter:** If we do have some emotional charge about an event or a person after doing the forgiveness list work, we can decide to talk to our healers about it, do some ritual, or determine what action to take. If we suspect that a part of ourselves may be absent, we can write an imaginary letter to that soul part or create a creative prayer/request for that part to come home. The invitation here is to do this as if you are trying to convince another person to return to a situation that was previously unsafe. What has changed in your life since these circumstances were present? Why would this part feel secure now when it didn't feel that way before?

Living Inspiration: Isa Gucciardi

I was introduced to Isa Gucciardi, Ph.D., through a mutual student and friend, Betty Jane Snow Wilhoit, who told me, "You two are up to the same things." Through our email correspondence, I came to agree; the Foundation of the Sacred Stream is a place where spiritual seekers and healers can find education and inspiration from a variety of spiritual traditions. I spoke with Isa Gucciardi regarding her work in the study and practice of soul retrieval.

GRS: Where do you personally see a hunger for the sacred the most?

IG: People will always look for alternatives when they have exhausted other pathways of understanding. I notice people will often turn to a spiritual path when they are suffering or see others suffering. This often widens their inquiry around spirit. When religious or healing institutions that are charged with providing care fail, it is also common for people to have a crisis of faith and see what else is out there.

GRS: How did the concept of soul retrieval come to be a vital part of your life and work? Why is it of value to you?

IG: Like other healers, I had a great deal of personal experience that I had difficulty understanding. I could not find the answers to what I was dealing with in conventional therapeutic models or in traditional forms of religion. This sent me on a quest. At a very young age, I became interested in alternative ways of looking at the world. My personal history included living in many cultures so I already had a broad range of inquiry. In pursuit of my quest for answers, I came across the concept of soul loss. When I heard the words, my ears perked up. I knew immediately, *that* was what I was suffering from. There had been no words before this that pointed to this experience at the core of my being.

After studying a lot of shamanic traditions academically, I began studying with Michael Harner and Sandra Ingerman. Sandra's book, *Soul Retrieval*, and her workshops had already clearly defined the concept of soul retrieval in the West. I worked with Michael as a medium for several years and became exposed to the kind of healing that was possible when working on the spirit level. I had also worked as a ground for a famous medium on the east coast and witnessed lots of spirit level healing through her work.

As it turns out, soul retrieval is a practice common to many shamanic traditions. I have found it helpful to study all the ways soul parts get separated from the mind-body complex of a person, place, or society. This has been a study I have been engaged in for almost twenty years through practicing and teaching Depth Hypnosis, which incorporates shamanic practice into its processes and practicing and teaching Applied Shamanism through the Foundation of the Sacred Stream. Applied Shamanism goes further than traditional shamanic practice in involving the client in all its processes—and the process of retrieving soul parts is no different. In Applied Shamanism, the client is encouraged to be active in integrating soul parts returned by the shamanic practitioner and is not just a passive bystander to the practitioner's efforts. Depth Hypnosis goes even further in involving the client in his or her own process of soul retrieval and power retrieval. Depth Hypnosis adopts the traditional methods of soul retrieval where the shamanic practitioner is doing most of the work and actually assists the client in becoming their own "shaman." This work is done by adapting the power retrieval process into a form of guided meditation—and by adapting the soul retrieval process into a hypnotherapeutic regression therapy process. When clients are more involved in their own healing, they do not have to be dependent on the practitioner for understanding. This is much more empowering than processes where the practitioner does all the "heavy lifting."

Soul loss is also happening on a larger scale on the entire planet. Soul loss is not limited to individual human experience. It is also quite evident that societies experience this. Examples of collective soul loss and its effects can be found by studying the experience of cultures, such as Native American cultures that have experienced genocide, or cultures in Africa where the demoralization generated by colonialism has created a cultural, political, and spiritual vacuum.

The Earth herself is in a state of soul loss due to the war that has been waged against her by unbridled industrialization. Even so, I have great faith in her regenerative capacity. There is much we can do as shamanic practitioners to heal, safeguard, and restore the Earth and the beings that dwell there. Working on a spirit level makes many things possible. So much that happens in spiritual reality affects material reality. It is important to remember this even though the effect of spiritual healing like soul retrieval may not always be immediately evident on a material level.

GRS: Why is soul retrieval important to our collective health?

IG: Of course, the collective is made of each individual. When individuals engage in soul retrieval on their own, it does affect the collective even if the individual is not aware of the collective. But when individuals participate in change with the collective in mind, miraculous things can happen. On the other hand, when you have many individuals who are experiencing soul loss or power loss on an individual level, the collective cannot help but demonstrate the experience of soul or power loss at the collective level.

Right now in the West and across the world, we have societal structures that are dependent on the perpetuation of power loss on the individual level. This is because most societal structures are set up so that they require the individual to give their personal power to the societal structure to maintain it. Sometimes the societal structures, such as education or industry, even demand soul parts of the individuals. This creates soul loss and power loss in each individual. This state of soul loss and power loss, which can look like self-doubt or feeling helpless, binds the individuals to the collective as they look to societal structures to remedy the sense of loss they experience. But it is a vicious cycle. The societal structures themselves only exist on the power and soul they have taken from the individuals, so they really have nothing to offer the individual. Indeed, as the individual looks to the society's structures for support, the society takes the opportunity to just take more power from them.

This is a terrible state of affairs that can only be remedied by returning each individual to a state of wholeness through power retrieval and soul retrieval. When all individuals in a society are whole, the collective will be whole and integrated.

GRS: What are the side effects of a world where people don't understand or value soul retrieval?

IG: The side effect is an entire world experiencing soul loss. That is what we are living in right now, on a planetary, societal, familial, individual, and environmental level. We can't even recognize what it is or what it arises from, which makes it very difficult to heal. People don't understand the consequences of pulling power from "easy" negative power sources like hatred and greed to remedy the state of soul loss they find themselves in. Pulling power from negative sources actually causes and exacerbates soul loss. We really do need to understand the enormous downside of negativity from this point of view. His Holiness the Dalai Lama is not kidding when he says that the cultivation of compassion is the salvation of the planet.

GRS: What do you see as the major barriers to including these practices in the world we live in?

IG: The biggest barrier is that the current scientific imperialism existing in modern thought precludes the concept of spirit and the unseen. We are addicted to the scientific method to measure ridiculous things, such as the hair growth of a mouse under certain conditions. I cannot deny that good things can come with the scientific method but it can also be used as a sledgehammer. It is shortsighted to believe that if something is not replicable, it is not valid. The world of spirit will never fit those parameters. And the experience of spirit is valid, as any visionary will tell you. Many people can't understand or imagine the world of spirit because of the limitations of the scientific worldview they have been taught to adopt.

When illness is caused by the rending of the fabric of the spirit, it can't be healed by a model that does not recognize the existence of spirit. This is a great tragedy. It is actually unscientific to preclude a whole area of experience out of hand. Including the world of spirit would allow people to have access to the power of soul retrieval to heal illnesses that are not originating on a physical level at all.

GRS: What do you think would change in the world if soul retrieval became integrated in our culture or available within our systems of medicine? For instance, what would be altered if medical practitioners included the referral for soul retrieval as an option in their recommendations for the treatment of illness?

IG: From a shamanic perspective, all illness is caused by soul loss, power loss, and energetic interference. Modern medicine is only dealing with imbalance when it appears on a physical and mental level. Shamanic practice recognizes that illness at the spirit level will move to the emotional level if it is not addressed. If it is not addressed at the emotional level, it moves to the mental level. If it is not addressed at the emotional level, it moves to the physical level, where it is generally harder to ignore. Modern Western medicine practitioners are picking up a problem long into its evolution when they only treat physical symptoms. Many events have already led to that physical symptom. Because shamanic practice is always focused on healing the spirit, it addresses the symptom at its point of origin no matter where on the spectrum it is manifesting.

In Huna, there is the concept of Ho'oponopono, which means making the situation right. When shamanic practitioners are called to perform healing on a physical level, they ask that the person receiving the healing enter a process of intense inquiry into the unseen aspects of their relationships with other people through the processes of Ho'oponopono. This is because it is understood that the unseen plays a role in the development of disease. For instance, if a person has unresolved anger in a relationship with a family member, this can contribute to the manifestation of physical disease from a shamanic point of view. The processes of Ho'oponopono seek to address and resolve the anger in order to weaken the effect the anger has on the physical disease. Physical healing does not even begin until these corrections are addressed. I think that Western doctors could actually benefit from working with this method, especially for those patients who are not responding positively to other forms of treatment.

However, what we see these days is that everyone wants to take a pill because they don't want to have to take responsibility for their experience. The Western system is set up for the doctor to take responsibility for their patient's experience. If things go wrong, it is the doctor who did not heal the person adequately. Doctors think they like this system because it creates more power for them, and patients think they like it because they are not required to take responsibility. If the treatment doesn't work, they simply search for a better doctor. If people were sent into a soul retrieval process, it is possible that they would heal more deeply and fully because they would be required to look more fully at their experience. In Depth Hypnosis, we understand that the symptom is the teacher and we ask it what it has to say. In Western medicine, practitioners and patients are out to kill the symptom, not to listen to it.

GRS: What is your offering to these interesting times in terms of your work?

IG: My offering is certainly not what I expected it was going to be. My quest in the beginning of my healing journey was to understand my own issues. Because I had a lot of issues, I had a long quest. In an effort to heal myself of imbalance that was untouched by traditional Western methods, I had to look deeply within myself and beyond the world of the rational. As I healed myself, I gathered many tools. When I decided to work with those tools with others, I realized I had developed a good foundation for the work that channeled through me as I continued in my quest to understand imbalance in others. Over the course of ten years, the body of work that we teach at the Foundation of the Sacred Stream came to me in study, meditation, and straight-ahead channeling sessions. The centerpiece of this work is Depth Hypnosis, which combines shamanism, Buddhism, transpersonal psychology, energy medicine, and hypnotherapy. Depth Hypnosis uses hypnosis to alter a waking state of consciousness. This model uses the constructs of shamanism, such as soul retrieval and power retrieval, and incorporates Buddhist understandings regarding the nature of suffering. We guide clients to their own sources of soul loss. The clients discover what this is for themselves. This is very different from traditions where the shaman does all the work. We don't use drums or plants to alter consciousness. We use hypnosis. In an altered state, the client follows the presenting symptoms to find the source of imbalance driving the symptoms. More often than not, the source of the symptom is a form of soul loss. The client is guided to bring the soul part back and help reintegrate it into their larger experience through soul retrieval processes, which are adapted into the hypnotherapeutic process.

In my first year of practice, I had a longer waiting list of clients than I could possibly treat and so I began to teach what I knew to others in an effort to help everyone who was asking for help. As I sought to convey everything I could, I realized my students needed more training in each of the components that make up Depth Hypnosis. I started with teaching Depth Hypnosis, and then added Applied Shamanism, Integrated Energy Medicine, and Buddhist Psychology. Then I developed a program of Transpersonal Studies to help people begin to perceive the events of their lives as moments on their paths of spiritual inquiry and discovery. In the Destination Studies program, students come to different places on the Earth where different wisdom traditions originated as the peoples who lived there listened to what the Earth was saying in each place. Through the shamanic journey, we are able to access those teachings in a fresh way and touch not only the wisdom held in each place, but also honor and respect those who accessed them first.

The offerings from the Foundation of the Sacred Stream are an enormous body of work. The Sacred Stream Center has been an incubator for other teachers and artists who are developing their own work in the world. Through all of our activities, we are engaged in the creative and dynamic process of cultivating and encouraging the processes of consciousness.

GRS: What does the world/what do humans need most right now in order to return to healthy culture?

IG: The main thing humans need to do is take responsibility for themselves. People have gone to sleep in order to pretend they don't have to deal with things that they have to deal with. They would rather take a pill or numb out than understand why they are hurting. What is needed right now is education. I am dedicated to education. I firmly believe that if people understand the full consequences of their actions, they would make different choices. If they could have resources and tools to develop themselves, I believe that they would do so.

CHAPTER SEVEN

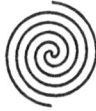

Personal Practice:
When We Practice Presence

Submit to a daily practice.
Your loyalty to that
is a ring on the door.
Keep knocking, and the joy inside
will eventually open a window
and look out to see who's there.

— RUMI

N early every morning, I light a candle and sit in meditation. Sometimes I write on a piece of paper what the intention is that I would like to set for the day and place it underneath the candle. My practices change seasonally and vary over the years. Sometimes I do cleansing work, changing the quality of my own breath to change my mood or attitude. Sometimes I do a yoga sequence or take a walk or write morning pages in my journal for 20 minutes. Sometimes I sing and imagine my heart opening to the work I am meant to do in the world. Sometimes I pray for people who have been affected by the most recent disaster, picturing the faces I have seen on the internet news *and asking how I can help. I often see the faces of my patients, friends or family and receive insight about the experiences that they have shared with me. My daily practice teaches me what is mine to create or destroy each day and overall in our collective journey toward health.*

∞

"I feel lost, fearful, and depressed, like I don't know who I am or why I'm here," my forty-seven-year-old patient reveals when I ask him about his mood. I ask him about personal practice, anything that he does that can help him remember himself. He talks about how running used to help him feel connected but he had to stop because of a knee injury. I tell him that we can work on relieving knee pain in our acupuncture sessions, but wonder if there is another activity that he can use to reconnect with a sense of purpose or connection, or at least, curiosity. He mentions how relaxed he felt when he listened to the chanting of the Buddhist monks when he did some work in Tibet. He decides to listen to a recording of their chanting daily to inspire him to chant along with them or on his own.

Sacred Exploration:

Personal practice lays a foundation for something greater than our unremitting daily schedules even if it is just a deepening or opening into your body in the present moment. This is a template of an action that holds an intention. Doing these practices habitually, even daily, keeps our emotions and even the pieces of our souls firmly anchored in embodied life experience. Yoga, prayer, meditation, exercise, dance, tai chi, martial arts, breathing methods, chanting, playing music, art, cooking and writing are all examples of regular personal practices. The choices are infinite.

"A practice is a habit we have chosen," Joanna Macy reminds us. We have the complete authority and choice to integrate practices, which carry our healing intentions and visions for ourselves, our clients, our patients, and our planet, into our daily lives.[1] Personal practice helps us find our way back to the core of who we are. Throughout time, people have used a ritual or regular activity to make a connection to the source of their spirituality whether this is Love, Goddess, God, Spirit, Nature, or something else. The repetitive nature of this practice is what makes it useful. Routine is a word that we often associate with a lackluster life or boredom. However, in this case, it is routine that speaks to the body, mind, and spirit in a language that they can understand. The ritual of personal practice can communicate to our complicated bundle of bones, neurochemistry, and muscles even when our minds are spinning madly and stress hormones are flowing liberally.

Personal practice establishes a baseline for sanity to shift out of difficult sensations and emotions. Just doing the practice helps us to relax or remember goals that we have set for our well-being. It can be a reminder for us to return to presence, no matter what is happening in our thoughts. It can tear us away from past regrets and future worries. A chance to be in the now.

We are overwhelmed with data and information. Most of us cannot mentally process the level and frequency of stressors that we endure on a daily basis. We know that stress becomes lodged in our body, our soma, to be dealt with at a later time. But when? A regular practice can become that time to clear the decks. Our practices remind us how we want to act, and allow us to create some space outside of reaction so that we can learn to respond to things more holistically.

One purpose of emotions is to get our attention and tell us something is really important. But in a fast paced world, emotions often overwhelm us. We spend time feeling triggered by situations in the present that remind us of the past. These emotional triggers can hijack the body, infusing us with stress hormones and clouding our problem-solving skills. We are literally stuck in the past, experiencing trauma that is not happening in the moment. Our practice can be a strategy to release this state of fight, flight, or paralysis and give us access to our whole being again. I think of it as a miniature form of soul restoration and a visit to my creative brain.

In modern technological culture, our attention is in demand on multiple fronts. Study after study shows that multitasking does not increase our ability to pay attention to stimuli. We cannot integrate information without time and repeated experience. However, knowing that doesn't change the fact that we are expected or asked to attend to various factors simultaneously. I often catch myself with two computer monitor screens with nine windows open and talking with someone on the phone about a collaborative project deadline, which is maybe even unrelated! If my breath has climbed up into my chest and I notice that I feel anxious, I stand up, close my eyes, drop my breath into my belly or the sides of my ribs. I might drink water or herbal tea, look at something beautiful or take a break or a walk. Getting embodied is always a useful practice, wherever you are.

We can pretend to thrive in this non-stop, hyperactive environment and some may even keep this appearance up for a long stretch, but the evidence shows another pattern. Over time, we lose our ability to give attention to ourselves, our bodies, our relationships. We no longer have time to develop any kind of wisdom or long term memory, only to fill our brains with even more data. This is a pattern that leads to both disease and the inability to consider the impact of our actions. We are simply moving too fast to attend to anything.

Relieving stress is not a necessary component of personal practice, but it is often something that we combine with it, out of necessity. Some people relax by getting quiet in their bodies or environment, finding stillness in some way. Others tend towards a more active practice that allows them to release tension and unwind afterwards. It is unlikely that we will have an ecstatic experience every time we go to the gym or pick up our journal. With the dedication of time and energy, however, we have the chance to touch something beneath the surface of ourselves or shift an emotional state that is preventing us from seeing a bigger perspective. Perhaps many humans need a habitual doorway to some form of the sacred in order to thrive.

Personal practice can become our foundation on which to build a life that includes the things we want. Repetition brings mastery and as humans, we long to master something and claim expertise. However, the word practice keeps us humble, implying that we will not ever reach the pinnacle but that we will return again and again to seek improvement, reconnection. We can take time to remember ourselves, our intentions, our wildest dreams, and the truth of who we are. Doing this will improve our personal health, and it is hard to imagine that a population of people who are taking responsibility for returning to who they really are would not help our relationships with each other.

One of the largest barriers that people express is finding the time to do their practice. If this is an obstacle, perhaps our definitions of personal practice could become more imaginative. My friend, Dawn has often said to me that she sees a lot of folks who are parents and don't have a personal practice because of the amount of time that parenting demands. She often says, "Don't your children deserve to see a parent who values a personal practice?" Where could the time fit? Could it be done together as a family?

Complicated practices can be beautiful, but sometimes, less is more. I tell my professional development clients and patients, "The best and most effective kind of regular personal practice is the one you will actually do." What is the simplest and most effective routine that could be incorporated into your life with the intention of bringing you back to yourself?

Revolutionary Healing Dares:

I dare you to find a personal practice that you can actually do every single day OR keep doing the one that you know works for you. I dare you to make it simple, achievable, and authentic, something that provokes the sacred within you. I dare you to give yourself permission to forget or fall out of the practice and then bring it back into your life when you notice that you have done so. I dare you to connect to what matters, to connect to what is at your core. I dare you to ask someone else what matters deeply to them and to remind them to visit the core of themselves on a regular basis. I dare you to tell someone that you care about what matters deeply to you.

Spiritual Inventory:
Exercises for Personal Practice

1. **Identify your practice:** What is one activity you can do with the intention of setting aside a regular opening for yourself to practice presence? Remember that you can include elements of Embodiment, Connection to Land, Alchemy, Ritual, Creativity, Ecstasy, or Soul Restoration in your practice. Also, remember that simple is best! You can choose from these examples or create your own: meditation (sitting or walking/moving), yoga, breathwork, cooking, painting, dancing, chanting, playing or listening to music, laughing, walking, running, another kind of exercise, writing, reading, mindfulness in some form, sculpting, creating any kind of art, gardening, singing, cleaning, praying,

tai chi, reading or writing poetry, knitting, sewing, yard work, carpentry, martial arts, playing games, taking herbs or vitamins, hiking or working with dreams.

2. **Calendar therapy:** Block out non-negotiable time on your calendar to do this practice. Ideally, this is every day but if that is not a possibility, set it aside with regularity. Often, if it is on our calendar, it will happen! If you do not have the time right now, choose a time in the next month when you will begin this practice.

3. **Personal Practice buddy:** Find someone else who enjoys this practice or just someone who is willing to encourage you or ask you how it is going. When we have support in our endeavors, we are more likely to succeed!

Living Inspiration: Dawn Isidora

I sat with my friend, colleague, and coconspirator, Dawn Isidora, in her home in Portland, Oregon. Dawn's extensive background is rooted in hypnotherapy and Earth-based spirituality. She has many years of experience as a professional dancer, deeply intuitive workshop leader, and Kundalini yoga teacher that inform her private practice where she provides spiritual mentorship and counseling.

GRS: Where do you personally see a hunger for the sacred the most?

DI: I notice people falling prey to compartmentalizing their lives. They are yearning to have that sensation of connection to spirit throughout all parts of their lives, in their work, their relationships, in their daily interactions and not just squirreled away to be taken out at holidays, special ceremonies, or even weekly services. People want to feel that their lives are connected and meaningful all the time. In my mentorship practice, a lot of people, maybe even the majority of my clients, come to me because they are trying to manifest that sensation of spirit in their lives more tangibly. They are experiencing a lack of the sacred, a lack of that kind of connection.

GRS: How did personal practice come to be a vital part of your life and work? Why is it of value to you?

DI: I suppose it was a combination of things. I had tried a lot of things in searching for my own connection to Spirit. A dear friend, Thorn Coyle, really stresses the value of daily practice, and the more I explored that, the more truth I found there. In my spiritual mentorship practice, I have developed the idea a bit further. I've found that personal practice is most helpful when it has these five aspects: something physically active, like walking or yoga; something still, like meditation or silent prayer; something energetic, like chakra alignment or running life force energy; something inward gazing, like journaling or dreamwork; and some form of gratitude practice, reading poetry to that which you experience as divine or recounting all the things you feel grateful for.

The daily-ness of my practice is good for me. Finding those things that remind me of the way I am in the universe and remind me of how that feels and how I move through the world. I found my personal practice through trial and error. I have practices that I come back to over and over, so when I slip into a less desirable mode of being, I can call my practices back in my memory or do them and realign. I ask myself, how do I want to feel right now? Then I try to do what it takes to get myself there.

GRS: What is your personal practice these days?

DI: Before I answer that, I want to stress that my children are grown. I am self-employed and work out of my home. Because I work in the field of spiritual awareness, I feel it is especially important that I remain as clear as I possibly can. All this is to say, I don't want readers to feel overwhelmed. My practice works for me and my life. It's very important for folks to develop the practices that work for them and their lives.

When I first awake in the morning, I spend some time noticing what my dreams were, what images, sensations, impressions linger. Sometimes I write them down; sometimes I just spend some minutes in that liminal space, looking inward. Later in the morning, after the rest of the house has headed out into their day, I'll do my yoga set ending with a meditation period. I see clients in my home office during the day, so in addition, I practice a cleansing ritual for emotions and frustrations that arise in me that I may want to change. I use this ritual as one might use hand-washing. I do it in between clients to clear and reset. Late afternoon can be a harried or lower energy time of day for me, so just before I start fixing dinner,

I do my gratitude practice, recounting and naming all the things I can think of that I am grateful for that day, always including the beautiful food I have at hand to fix for my family, and then I run life force energy. I also take a walk on most days. Oftentimes, it's just a quick stroll around the block, but I make a point of noticing the elements without and within, greeting my tree friends, noticing the incremental changes as the wheel turns through the seasons. In addition, I have rituals and prayers around tending my altar spaces, cleaning the house, tending the garden, even taking a shower! When I list it out like this it sounds like a lot, but at this point, it's so integrated that I don't even notice. It has just become how I do things.

GRS: Why is the concept of personal practice important to our collective health?

DI: When you really buy in, as I do, to the concept that we are a part of a whole, it's important that each cell be healthy in order for the whole to be healthy. The whole cannot be healthy if it's made out of unhealthy parts. It's just math.

GRS: And so by doing personal practice, we add to the natural holism of humanity?

DI: Our own health is a part of the communal health; the part we have the most control over. There also seems to be the part that is harder to quantify—beyond how we feel physically or what we can measure physiologically through CT scans and PT scans. There have been studies that show that prayer is effective for healing, but no one understands exactly how. No one has been able to prove scientifically why or how acupuncture works but those of us who use it know that it does work; it helps us feel better.

It stands to reason that the energy we put out, the mood, actions, and behaviors that come from us, impacts the world. It is not just that we make the cell that is ourselves healthy, our relative sense of ease or dis-ease also impacts the cells that we come into contact with physically, spiritually, emotionally, however we are interacting with them.

GRS: What are the side effects of a world where people don't value personal practice?

DI: It ends up looking like a lot of shame inside ourselves and blame of others. At least that is the middle stage of the consequences; the end result is more dire. When we don't have a real and tangible experience of who we are, how we move through the world, and what our actual responsibilities are, the natural human response is to feel shame that we are not doing all we should or could or might be doing. Alternatively, we blame others for not living up to our expectations or what we think they should or could be doing. It is a vicious cycle.

I equate our personal responsibility to ourselves and the other beings in our family and community with Earth, one of the four sacred elements, along with Air, Fire, and Water that can lead to a strong link with Spirit. Earth is all about relationships. That is all that ecosystems are, simply systems of connections. People experience isolation in their lives, especially if they are in a shame and blame cycle. Personal practice would bring the sensation of connection to themselves, their community, or Spirit so lack of personal practice can leave a wake of alienation.

GRS: What do you see as the major barriers to including these practices in the world we live in?

DI: Time. I hear from clients in my practice with great regularity that people feel far too stretched already to set aside time for a spiritual practice. Folks are booked solid; we keep ourselves very busy. Ironically, this frenetic pace can exacerbate our sense of isolation and then we choose downtime pursuits that numb us from our sense of isolation. We watch television, surf the web and social media sites and this gives a feeling of connection even though we are mostly tuning out rather than in. Conversely, when we invest in connecting with ourselves, using a portion of the time we spend soothing and numbing to really reconnect with ourselves, that is a gateway into cracking open the dilemma of not enough time.

There is also a confusion of what a personal practice can be. People second-guess and judge their own choices, telling themselves what they have decided to do is not creative enough or not giving themselves permission for their personal practice to be authentic. "I should be doing silent sitting meditation for forty minutes" is another way to shame ourselves. People underestimate the importance of intent in their personal practice. Many things done with intention can be functional daily practices. Even activities we do every day: walking, bathing, cooking, cleaning, drinking water, moving our bodies, if they are done with focused intention, can be examples of connective practice or presence.

GRS: In its healthy function, what does personal practice offer to folks?

DI: Firstly, it creates a solid platform to return to when we get thrown off balance. When we do something mindful every day that creates a grounded-ness or presence, we program ourselves to return. We are creatures of habit, when we walk a certain path every day, that path becomes a pattern in our being. If you picture a path through a field, that path gets worn and we can find it again, it creates ease for us. If every day we choose another path to get from one side of the field to another, it can be confusing. If there is a practice you have done every day, all you have to do is show up at the path and it is there before you, even in a crisis. Additionally, it builds strength: physically, emotionally, spiritually, so that fewer things feel like they are at crisis level. That sensation of crisis seems to play havoc on our adrenal system, which leaves us susceptible to more illness, injury, general fatigue, and emotional exhaustion (which in turn seems to move into chronic depression) than when our adrenal system is not stressed.

GRS: What do you think would change in the world if personal practice became integrated in our culture or available within our systems of medicine? For instance, what would be altered if people could choose to code the development of a personal practice as an important factor in their recommendations for the treatment of illness?

DI: I think our dependence on some medications and drugs would shift. There is a lot of money wrapped up in giving people pills to fix things when longer term changes in lifestyle or practice, while not as easy as popping a pill, could make equal or greater difference, without the side effects. We could feel more in charge of our own wellness; being more active in our wellness is very much in our best interest. It's really time for us to no longer allow ourselves to be passive receivers of treatments. When we program our belief systems to know that we are active participants in our own wellness, it's a stronger and more sustainable model.

CHAPTER EIGHT

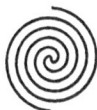

Shadow and Dreams:
The Stories Beneath the Stories

Sonnet XVII

I do not love you as if you were salt-rose, or topaz,
or the arrow of carnations the fire shoots off.
I love you as certain dark things are to be loved,
in secret, between the shadow and the soul.
I love you as the plant that never blooms
but carries in itself the light of hidden flowers;
...I love you because I know no other way...

— PABLO NERUDA

My lifelong struggle with an impulse to control my environment can sometimes manifest in arguments with those closest to me. I also hate to feel controlled by someone else and can react strongly to any perception that someone is trying to manipulate me, even if it isn't their intention. In many situations in my various workplaces, I have often been encouraged to take on more and more leadership roles; people say that they appreciate the way I take charge and lead a group to clear solutions. I worry that I am hiding the fact that I often take charge because I am attached to the outcome being positive and I want to have *a say in what happens. For a while, I attempt to ignore the "controlling" voice when it comes up in leadership situations. Instead, I pretend that I am laid back and able to go with the flow. Sometimes this works, but the controlling voice tends to get more insistent when I ignore it.*

A fantastic therapist suggests that this might be a shadow part of me, formed in service to some needs that I had in the past. She recommends that I be in dialogue with the part of myself that wants to be in charge all the time, to ask it what it wants. I do some journaling with the part of myself that I nicknamed the "Rigid Controller" or "RC" for short. I learn that this part of me had felt both ungrounded and out of control when I was growing up and never got to make choices about what happened to my body, mind and spirit. I remember that I had made a vow to never let that happen again once I was an adult. With this new information, I am more able to notice RC's voice when it comes up and listen to what is needed. I am often able to communicate my needs as requests and ask for feedback from my loved ones and coworkers. When I am in charge, I can say my piece and then ask others about what everyone else wants in the moment rather than going into an automatic response. This proves to be much more useful to my leadership and to my relationships.

∞

My 11 year-old client shares a dream in which he is on a ladder that scales a very large wall that holds thousands of cells. People live in these cells, very sparsely with a single bed and little furniture. I ask if the people can leave the cells or if they are kept there against their will. He responds that they came there by choice at first but now they are unable to leave. I ask him if this reminds him of anything in his life and he says, "Yes, it is like coming to live in America."

Sacred Exploration:

So much lies beneath the surface of our complex human natures. We keep secrets about our hopes, fears, dreams, and fantasies and sometimes refuse to share them with even our most intimate friends and partners. What is sacred or healthy about delving into these unknown, unchartered territories within ourselves?

Carl Jung coined the term 'shadow' to describe the unconscious impulses that often dictate our behavior and short-circuit our best intentions. Bringing these parts of ourselves into our awareness helps us integrate needs that we have ignored and gives us more freedom to choose our actions with integrity. The shadow is the part of the self that is hidden even from our own consciousness. Often it is hidden for fear that it would not be socially acceptable. For example, people commonly hide information about their sexual desires or proclivities so as not to experience rejection or ridicule.

Other times, parts of the self are hidden to protect the whole self from discomfort or disparity. For example, someone who had a childhood desire to be a performer but now works as a banker might experience discomfort when his cousin gets a role in a movie but not understand why. Bringing his childhood dream to be a performer to consciousness might have the consequence of making a change in his life. The shadow can act as an alarm clock, waking us to the pieces of our self that demand attention.

Developing awareness of the self and our own motivations is a prerequisite for many kinds of spiritual work. When we examine our projections and strong reactions to other people, we are able to reclaim the power and energy that we are giving to those projections. It makes sense that we would have greater ability to put our willpower behind the visions that we imagine if we were able to navigate around our obstacles to manifesting what we want.

Who is really in charge of our behavior? It is easy to blame others for "making" us do things. Advertising appeals to our primal needs in order to compel us to consume products. We are dissatisfied with our jobs but afraid of losing them so we do not take risks to improve our situations. We struggle in relationships, playing out our childhood fantasies and terrors and hoping that our partners can heal our wounds, becoming angry when they do not. We wish for a part of us who helps us make good decisions. Can I get a teacher, parent, leader or adult part of my personality, please?

Our subterranean needs employ the shadow parts of us are to make sure that these needs are met somehow. The shadow is expert at moving quickly so that the conscious parts of us are still scratching our heads and trying to decipher our own behavior. Patterns of addiction are perfect examples of this dialogue between our vision of who we want to be and the patterns of behavior that we exhibit. The addictive behavior may be a face of the shadow, asking for attention, showing us something yet to be heard.

Shame is a common response to our shadow-y behavior. The

trouble with shame is that it short-circuits the process and the need still does not get met, laying the ground for more shadow behavior in the future. When we make a mistake or act in a way that others find hurtful, if we simply say, "That wasn't like me," we don't get to hear what the underlying need was that fed our behavior. If we can shine the light into our subconscious and ask ourselves what part of us is not being fed, what need requires attention, we may be able to take responsibility for our behavior and meet our need in a more forthright way.

Sometimes irritation and envy can be clues to the needs of our shadow. Qualities that frustrate us when others exhibit them can show us parts that want to be integrated and reveal requirements that we didn't know we had. Carl Jung called this the negative shadow.[1] Qualities that we admire in others often signal untapped potential within ourselves. This is sometimes known as the "positive shadow." When we are attracted to or repelled by another, it is helpful to consider how we are similar to them or why their behavior affects us so strongly.[2]

One view of wholeness is that the shadow acts in service to us throughout our lives. Many times, in our families of origin, our self was created in a somewhat limited environment. It may have been necessary to relegate certain character traits to the shadows in order to survive. We may have had to gain the approval of our parents and other authority figures. As we evolve and find our own identities, those parts in exile see an opening to come back to the whole self. These rejected parts, according to Carl Jung, also hold amazing creative power.[3]

Understanding the shadow is a tool for us to learn from our mistakes and defenses, not to justify intolerable behaviors. It is different to have thoughts about hurting someone than to actually act abusively toward them. If we are the ones who act hurtfully, it is the moral thing to apologize and repair relationships. Sometimes we are the ones who have been wronged. Certainly, the shadow can overtake someone and cause people to act harmfully towards others. Removal of ourselves or other beings from harm would be the first step in the process. I believe that we can philosophize about the shadow, find compassion, and look at redemption or forgiveness for others but only after we have ensured that the damaging actions have stopped. This includes physical harm, emotional abuse, psychological threat and other situations where someone's health and well-being are at risk.

The shadow of our culture is something else to consider when we look at health care and where we are headed. Who does the current system benefit? Who suffers? What needs are we ignoring or not attended to? What negative effects of our current way of life on the larger body of our planet do we see?

When we get into a dialogue with the shadow, we open to the possibility of finally meeting our own needs, freeing up the emotional energy bound up in the shadow. This is a kind of alchemy. This holds true in a cultural context as well. Perhaps our collective development of this current system served a purpose for some time and we are in a different time now.

If we are able to discover the reasons for our behavior and shift out of our cycles of shame, we can integrate the pieces of our culture we have denied. When this happens, perhaps a visionary change can be made that considers a larger number of beings. We don't have to be perfect to be effective. We don't have to blame ourselves for participating in unhealthy systems set up without our approval; our responsibility is to change them dramatically. Our obligation is to create new ways of being that serve the health and happiness of all beings.

Many studies suggest that we do not use our brains to their full capacity. We do not use the wholeness of ourselves that is available to us. Each of us is a multifaceted creatrix, capable of splendor and terror. Acknowledging that there are multiple pieces of ourselves does not mean we are hearing voices. Our ability to develop a strong sense of our core and enter into conversation with all aspects of ourselves can lead us to better overall health.

The need to do things "right" can create uncomfortable feelings when other parts of us speak up and want to do things a different way. There is a tension between what feels good and what social expectations ask of us. A well-integrated person is able to listen to all parts of the self and negotiate a consensus, or at least a compromise. Sometimes there are parts of ourselves that do not quickly rise to our consciousness, making it necessary to seek to know them in other ways. We are enticed to explore the subconscious, the mysterious parts of ourselves, and the world of our dreams.

The understanding and interpretation of dreams is a pursuit that is shared worldwide. Dreams come from the deepest creative reaches of the body, mind and spirit and have universal messages to share. Many mystery traditions value the lessons that come to us under the cover of night, using our fears and desires to gain our attention and pass on these teachings. Dream work is another way that we can get information and messages from the parts of ourselves that are not the closest to our conscious mind. Sleep studies say that every human dreams even if we cannot remember the dreams upon waking. Many spiritual traditions have a long-standing practice of dream interpretation, including ancient Celtic religions and Sufism. Dreams were seen as gifts from the divine, the body, or spirits offering important messages.

Jung gave us the important language of archetype, a universal symbol that illustrates our collective unconsciousness. There can be subtle nuances to the way cultures interpret an archetype but they are fairly consistent, even when taken across borders and time. Archetypes go beyond our personal experience, for instance, the archetype of mother transcends any positive or negative interpretation we have of our own mothers. When we tap into the archetypal energy of mother, we include everything that makes the essence of "mother energy," and not another kind of energy. There would certainly be different interpretations of "mother" and "father" if this question was answered by people across different cultures, but there would be many similarities as well. During dream interpretation, Jung used to look at dream symbols in terms of archetypes. If his patient dreamed about a dog, he would ask how is a dog unlike any other animal, what is unique about a dog? Because dreams speak in the language of symbol and archetype that is both unique to the dreamer's subconscious and connected to the human collective consciousness, these questions are useful to decode dreams.

Jeremy Taylor is a skilled dream worker and author in California and a wonderful facilitator of processes he has designed to use in dream groups. These are valuable tools for the healing practitioner as well. Some of his principles are:

All dreams speak a universal language and come in the service of health and wholeness.

Only the dreamer can say with any certainty what meanings the dream may have.

There is no such thing as a dream with only one meaning.

No dreams come just to tell you what you already know.

When talking to others about their dreams, it is both wise and polite to preface your remarks with words to the effect that "if it were my dream…" and to keep this commentary in the first person as much as possible.[4]

Nightmares are a particular kind of dream, perhaps a message urgently vying for our attention in a jungle of stimuli. Our bodies have evolved to pay attention to things that cause adrenaline to flow. In our past, this might have been the approach of a predator. These days, it is more likely to be a third cup of coffee, a traffic jam, or a prolonged conflict with our supervisor, partner or children. What chance would a dream that brings a gentle message have of truly getting our attention? Nightmares are designed by our body, mind and spirit to override the competition and ask us to pay attention to something that needs to give us notice. Recurring dreams are sometimes the only way that our psyches can get in touch with us.

Like dreams, the shadow parts of us are often created in service. They may have been defense mechanisms or forms of protection. Often, their job was to keep us "safe" from harm, rejection, abuse or other negative experiences. We bump up against them when we take steps to achieve a goal or take more responsibility in our lives. It is common that the hidden parts of us prefer to stay with the status quo. They know changes upset the equilibrium in a way that might ultimately move us toward our dreams. If we move into a different phase of our lives, the shadow can feel threatened and potentially fear for its own survival.

The shadow part of us does not like the risk of exposure that we take when we accept more leadership, begin to grow intimate in a relationship, or start a new venture. The shadow can rear its head in many ways and its motivations may seem mysterious. Why would any part of ourselves want to sabotage our good intentions to fulfill our fondest desires for our lives? Like frightening dreams, our shadow is attempting to come in service, to remind us of unfinished work or forgiveness that we still need to offer ourselves from the past.

The unconscious will never be fully understood by the rational mind. Doing this work keeps us honest with ourselves and accountable to our relationships with others. Knowing ourselves better, even the parts of us that we would not show to the world, leads us towards wholeness. Self-awareness lessens the chances that we will act publicly in ways that don't support our visions of integrity and health. Then, we welcome the gifts from our subterranean impulses and our dreams into our lives to engage in discovery.

Revolutionary Healing Dares:

I dare you to embrace what lies in the shadows of your soul, begging to be included. I dare you to invite your nightmares to tea, thank them very much, and ask them what they want you to know. I dare you to shine a loving light on someone else's shadow, to humanize their faults and make room for their mistakes and therefore your own. I dare you to illuminate the collective shadow of our health care, speak about what is not working and make new choices for yourself, your loved ones, and this planet. I dare you to remember your dreams and ask other people about their dreams to elucidate the unseen world from which so much wisdom arrives.

Spiritual Inventory:
Exercises for Shadow and Dreams

1. **Dream Journal exercise:** Write down your dreams. Keep a dream journal next to your bed and record anything you can remember about your dreams as soon as you wake. With practice, you will recall more and more detail. Share your dreams with someone. Jeremy Taylor talks a lot about how to start a dream group based on his principles of dreamwork. Consider reading his work or trying it out for yourself.

2. **Shadow identification:** Who is the person who irritates or upsets you the most? What is it that is so frustrating about them? Are they possibly showing you an unclaimed quality or potential about yourself?

   Who is the person whom you admire most? What is remarkable about this person? Are they possibly showing you an unclaimed potential or quality about yourself?

3. **Nightmares or disturbing dreams:** Find a place to sit with your journal. Choose the most provocative character in your dream and ask them: What do you want? Why did you come? Why this dream now? Write in your journal from the perspective of that dream figure and answer those questions. You may also ask if there is anything else that you need to know right now.

4. Shadow parts revealed: What is your most commonly used defense mechanism when you are upset and feel trapped? What does your reactive state look or sound like? What stories or beliefs run through your head? When was the first time you remember feeling this way?

It can sometimes be good to look at these reactive states as characters that we play, as if in the movies. If your defensive personality had a name, what would it be? What would this part of you look like? What is its job in your life?

Living Inspiration: Anne Hill

Anne Hill, D.Min. is a brilliant and grounded writer, educator, dreamworker, and consultant. She teaches and speaks about dreams and spirituality, coaches authors and thought leaders on content strategy, and hosts a video interview series on dreams. A lifelong Bay Area resident, she lives in Bodega Bay and holds a black belt in aikido. We sat together in Oakland and discussed the influence of dreams, even the scary ones, on our collective health.

GRS: Where do you personally see a hunger for the sacred the most?

AH: It comes up a lot in the dream groups that I lead, but I see it even more often in my coaching practice in the professional world; I see it in people who are trying to build their platform and express their life's work. I see it all the time. I shouldn't be surprised, but I still have to remind myself to go beyond the compartmentalization in my own mind that some people are into spirituality and others are focused on business. I can never assume that someone who comes to me for one thing isn't actually looking for the other. For example, many of my dreamwork clients are actually dealing with work or career issues and we move into coaching. We know that dreams bridge the left and right brain hemispheres and the different parts of our lives, so it's actually a perfect merging of modalities.

GRS: Have you had to do work around your own compartmentalization to integrate what you present?

AH: Going off the beaten path so much in my career, I've had to trust my own dreams when they say I am headed in the right direction, that I am not making a huge mistake, that all my leaps of faith are worth it. The voice that says it's not going to work turns out to be my fear talking. This perspective is exactly what people are hungry for, so I'm grateful for all the moments of doubt I've had to overcome along the way.

GRS: How did work with dreams become a vital part of your life?

AH: I started writing down my dreams as a teenager. Then when my kids were in preschool I was part of a women's book group with a few of the other moms from the preschool. One month we read Jeremy Taylor's book on group dreamwork and decided to try it for a summer. To make a long story short, eighteen years later we still meet almost every week to share our dreams, and four out of seven of us are original members of the group!

Having that outlet, especially as a young mother, has really helped me reflect on and integrate all of my life experiences. I did not associate dreamwork with spiritual work at first; I had it compartmentalized. At one point, I noticed that doing dreamwork activated the same parts of my brain that got activated when I did ritual or trance work. I had to take a look at my assumptions: actually, dreamwork was a valuable resource that I had been pigeonholing as a means of psychological insight. The other cool thing is that my dream group has now been going on far longer than any spiritual group I've been in.

Dreams are an amazing teacher about the slow process of change. The human pace for creating deep, lasting change is just glacial. For instance, I had dreams ten to fifteen years before my divorce that predicted exactly what would happen, but at the time if someone had said, "Hey, I think you need to look at your relationship," it would not have felt true at all. If I look back at those dreams, though, there is a popcorn trail. It takes ten years to make a change, even longer sometimes. That has changed my perception of ritual and the weekend workshop culture. It takes much longer to fully make a life change.

GRS: How is dreamwork important to our collective health?

AH: The more we can access our underlying motivations and inspirations, the clearer our actions will be. That is fundamental. My goal in dreamwork is to help people find their true north. What is the most important thing for you? Where do you find beauty? Dreams are so good at showing us images of incredible awe-inspiring beauty. If I can get to that place with people, the moment in a dream where beauty emerges, that is the core, where our soul is finding resonance, integration, and alignment in profound ways. My job is to keep pointing to that.

It's long-term stuff. The older I get, the more of a Taoist I become. I would love to say that this is going to change the world, but honestly who knows? It certainly eases the suffering in that moment in the world, gives people tools to recreate and anchor to the beauty that comes from within them. I am less attached to outcome these days, but even more passionate about facilitating those moments of clarity.

In the collective, we are going through a Plutonian phase; I like the idea that Pluto creates addition through subtraction. Things get stripped away and we get down to the core. That is going on in a big way for those I come in contact with. Let's focus on letting go, making room for grace.

GRS: What are the side effects of a world where people don't value their dreams?

AH: Dreams are like the pancreas. You can live your life without knowing where the pancreas is or what it does, but if it starts acting up, you get a crash course on the pancreas and it really hurts. The dreaming function, bringing the subconscious into conscious awareness, is just part of how our mind works. It is a system of our body. A lot of people don't remember their dreams, but they wake in the morning with the answer, the solution, the intervention. That's the process I want to help people understand, before they reach a pain point. We need a way for our unconscious needs and impulses to come into the daylight or else they really can bite you.

GRS: What would change if dreamwork were integrated into health care?

AH: A friend of mine who is an MD had a patient who told her about a dream of a tattered butterfly landing on her neck, barely alive. My friend thought, "Let's test her thyroid," which is a butterfly-shaped gland at the base of the throat. Sure enough, she had hypothyroidism. Dreams are giving us health information all the time; having some proficiency in dreams or at least a thumbnail sketch of the symbolism and process of dreaming would be immensely helpful for practitioners. Think of pediatricians: children have such an active dream life. It could be a place to really tap into what is going on.

GRS: What is your offering to the world through this work?

AH: I was trained by Jeremy Taylor, such a wise and generous man, and a founder of the grassroots dreamwork movement. I do less self-help and psychology these days. I am interested in dreams that go in a spiritual direction. I want to emphasize beauty, reaffirm spiritual connection, and help people rebuild trust in their own intuition. Dreamwork is not solely the tool of the priest or the scientist; we can all use it as a tool of "the commons." I want to move away from only fixing the broken and help people support what is good.

GRS: What does the world need right now to return to collective health?

AH: It feels like many things are falling apart on a grand scale. If we can fall without fear, that is a good thing. I once had this dream of falling from an airplane, and had that terrible sensation of vertigo and nausea. And then I had a semi-lucid moment within the dream and my aikido training kicked in. I wondered, "If I were on the ground right now, what would my stance be?" I got into my aikido stance and suddenly the ground rose gently up to meet my feet. I might still be falling but if I'm centered, it doesn't matter where I am. Anything we can do to dial back the fear is helpful. Fear is our worst enemy right now.

GRS: What is your personal practice around dreamwork these days?

AH: Dreamwork has become intricately woven into my daily practice over the past twenty years. I don't write down my dreams every night. But I do try to get seven to eight hours of sleep most nights, so that even if I don't remember them I know I am getting the benefits of enough dreaming sleep. I believe that if we miss recording a night's dreaming (or a week, or even a month), whatever important messages those dreams held will be repeated for our benefit when we are ready to pay attention again. And, meanwhile, like our pancreas, they are just working in the background to keep us healthy.

I carry vivid or troubling dream images around with me as I go through the day, reflecting on the emotional states embedded in the image and feeling my way into correlations with my waking life experience. It's kind of like keeping a jigsaw puzzle piece in your hand all the time, until you finally find that unexpected spot where it fits perfectly. Just today I had an aha moment about a brief dream snippet I've been thinking about from last month, and realized that the figures in my dream actually represent the businesses I have started in my life.

Sometimes we get to this material through talking dreamwork, but unless you are working with a seasoned group it can stay pretty mental and not get into the physical, emotional, and spiritual dimensions of your dreams. This "lucid waking" technique is a profound somatic practice. I am certainly not dreaming my way aimlessly through the day, but I am exercising that expanded awareness of holding both dreaming and waking states simultaneously.

The other times when I work actively on dreams by myself are during periods of wakefulness in the night and early morning. I will cast back in my mind for a feeling state or image from a dream, and hold it in my energy field. I breathe deeply, really relax into it, and stay there in meditation for several minutes letting my body and spirit talk to me. Sometimes nothing comes, and I drift back to sleep or decide to get up. Other times, I receive powerful insights that stay with me for years. The body knows so much, yet we rarely let it speak to us. This is one way I have found to correct that imbalance for myself.

GRS: What do you recommend others do if they want to work with their dreams?

AH: Dreamwork begins with cultivating healthy sleep habits. Beyond that, there is remembering dreams, and developing the habit of recording them. I suggest that everyone find at least one dream buddy, where part of your friendship is that you tell each other your dreams. Being in a dream group is fantastic practice, and there are so many excellent workshops to attend these days, too. Take advantage of all the videos and other online resources from dream experts, and don't be afraid to pick up random dream dictionaries as you're learning about your own dream meanings. You never know where you will find a morsel that really speaks to you.

I recommend that people start a somatic dream practice by holding deeply peaceful dream images within them during the day. Hold one image for a month and see what happens. These images are such a gift, and we often appreciate them for a day or two, and then set them aside to look for the next dream. This is a mistake. We need to appreciate all the gifts we are given, to receive the love and healing the dream is offering, and to allow ourselves to be held and transformed by the vast wisdom of our dreaming minds.

CHAPTER NINE

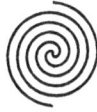

Alchemy: The Art of Changing a Life

Exercises on Themes from Life
Speaking of death
and decay
It hardly matters
Which
Since both are on the
way, maybe–
to being daffodils.

— ALICE WALKER

I am in a continuing education workshop where we are discussing Jung's shadow and its role in addiction. I scribble in my notebook: *"At the roots of all my shadow parts are potential gifts."*

My struggles with addiction, depression, and my own health provide me with empathy and insight into the healing processes of my patients. My desire to be in charge of my own life has transformed into leadership skills. My perfectionism leads me to write and teach work that inspires and touches others' lives. My hunger for a spirituality that is grounded in the earth pushes me to create sacred spaces wherever I am and advocate for places that need care. My fear and sorrow about *the state of the planet motivates me to action in its service. I realize that this is a kind of alchemy; all of my greatest struggles become my jewels, my ability to give back to the world.*

∞

A newly sober 27 year-old comes to get support for staying drug free. She is particularly mourning the way that cocaine made her feel more confident at parties and confessed to a lifetime of shyness. When asked what she most wants to change about herself, she replies that she would like to be able to speak with authority in the oral presentations that are part of her job. We talk about her discomfort in social situations and the desire to find her voice as being potential material for her to take through an alchemical process as she creates a new life without substances. She says, "I'm not sure that there could ever be anything positive about being an introvert but I'm willing to look at it."

Sacred Exploration:

How do we truly change? What is the process by which we can truly welcome all the pieces of ourselves into a whole person? Let's say you do it all. You stay present in your body and adopt a personal practice. You hike, take a painting class and create rituals to celebrate and mark changes. You call the lost parts of yourself home and start to recognize pieces you have hidden in shadow. Now you know yourself better, but when the going gets rough, you revert to acting the same old ways!

Isn't it more painful to be aware of our patterns if we seem to not be able to do anything differently? What moves self-discovery to action? How can we discover the essence of a characteristic about ourselves that drives us crazy and change it into something that expresses our true soul nature?

In many cultures throughout time, the answer would have been through alchemy. Alchemy is more than just an old wizard bent over a fire, brewing potions that can make gold out of lead. It's the precursor of modern chemistry, homeopathy and many contributions to modern medicine. Alchemy is a holistic view of change as transformation of a substance from one state to the next. The substance is affected by various processes along the way, but the basic properties of the substance remain the same, even at the end of the alchemical progression.

Alchemy is fundamentally different from the way we often approach change in modern culture. The principles of alchemy can be useful in changing our relationships to stories and situations that we believe to be our nemeses or our wounds. We try to rid ourselves of qualities or situations that we do not want and bring in or invite what we do want. This is a good idea, but, as we discovered in shadow work, many of the behaviors and stories that we don't like may be serving us in ways that we don't consciously understand. Let's say you want to change your anger issues so you breathe out irritation and breath in love as a meditation twice daily. But because the patterns of frustration were deeply ingrained to protect you and your younger siblings from a childhood caregiver's anger, they always return. The patterns have not been transmuted at the core so they persist. Healing in an alchemical sense means something different than out with the old, in with the new.

Alchemists would say that there is a gift hidden in the most difficult experiences of our lives. The Great Work of alchemy is to discover what these shining teachings are, to change our own lead into gold. In order to do this, the alchemists would take a personal story or a behavioral pattern through a series of processes. This story or pattern would be considered the Prima Materia (Latin for first material) with which the alchemist would work toward transmutation. Alchemy is the opposite of a disposable culture. Everything is of value.

In the world where we will use our medicine, we will see people at their point of crisis or breakdown. We can be responsible for assisting something new coming into being, but we as global revolutionary healers have to be willing to sift through the trash, sit in discomfort, and help code this crisis as a turning point. This can be quite uncomfortable; especially when we don't know what the outcome will be.[1]

A wise patient once said to me, "Health isn't always about going back to where you were." Often, people come to be fixed by whatever art we practice. The unspoken request is for the healer to "put me back to the way that I was" even if that way was not functional. As healers, we know that sometimes this is impossible and a transformation is needed for the person to grow. Using the principles of alchemy, we support people in changing perspective on their injury/illness and assist their transformation. Lorie Dechar, author, teacher, and alchemical acupuncturist, reminds us, "The decision not to restore but to move forward toward an unknown possibility was the beginning of Taoist alchemy."[2]

Another important characteristic of an alchemical process is that it cannot be consciously controlled. The alchemist may be able to choose the vessel and the lab and add substances to the Prima Materia or take it through experiments. Often, there is only patience and waiting to see what will happen. In metallurgy, this transformation happened in a laboratory and the substance or Prima Materia would be burned, dissolved, separated, and reformed. It would rot, ferment, and then be distilled and washed repeatedly. The Prima Materia would transmute over time, uncovering its true essence.

Alchemy begins with an archetypal descent, a change beyond our control or a reminder that something is not quite healed. Normal methods of soothing do not ease our dissatisfaction and we begin to suspect that a drastic change is required for our survival. The alchemist must be brave and also has to come to terms with the truth that there is no turning back.

In my weekend alchemy classes, I have people bring to the workshop a story or a pattern about themselves that they are interested in transforming. What we discover each time is that our most potent gifts and abilities have their roots in our most frustrating stories, our shameful coping mechanisms, and sometimes our wounds themselves. When we transform, it is from wound to wonder. James Hillman reminds us that our painful experiences become the source for the creation of our own soul journey: "We may imagine our deep hurts not merely as wounds to be healed but as salt mines from which we gain a precious essence and without which the soul cannot live. The fact that we return to these deep hurts, in remorse and regret, in repentance and revenge, indicates a psychic need beyond a mere mechanical compulsion...We make salt in our suffering and by working through our sufferings, we gain salt, healing the soul ...A trauma is a salt mine; it is a fixed place for reflection about the nature and value of my personal being, where memory originates and personal history begins. These traumatic events initiate in the soul a sense of its embodiment as a vulnerable experiencing subject."[3]

Through the lens of alchemy, the most beautiful trait in each of us is the core of our deepest pain. Painful memories of the past surface, not to torture us, but to signal us. We break them open and look inside them for their teaching. After an alchemical process, we might discover that having a sick parent may have granted us an increased sensitivity to how someone's body is feeling without that person telling us. Surviving childhood abuse may have given us the ability to "read" a room and know immediately what the mood is. No one chooses their childhood or past; we get what we get. Alchemists say that nothing is junk. What we dismiss as refuse is often the most potent Prima Materia of all.

We live in a world where everything is expendable. Rubbish is "thrown away" and we ship it to a landfill to slowly break down. When something breaks, many times, it will cost more to repair than to replace. Our materials are less expensive and the quality is also less desirable or the materials are made of something that causes cancer or will not easily biodegrade. Our physical and spiritual health care requires that this cultural attitude shift. A science of scavenging or recycling materials is needed on every level.

We must apply this alchemy to other people as well. Buddhism teaches us that we could pay the people who annoy and infuriate us as they are the best teachers about ourselves. If we have patience with this discovery process, we make different choices, and find more compassion for ourselves and the irritating people in our workplace or family. It is possible that we can use our own frustration with other humans as Prima Materia to look at our own buried potential.

In our larger culture, we are quick to toss away people or run from relationships, especially those who we don't get along with or those who frighten us. When people can't produce the behavior that we require, we often write them off as useless. Alchemy declares that our refugees, our homeless, addicts, our mentally ill, our disabled, and disenfranchised minorities have rare and hidden gold for our culture. What would have to change before we were willing as a culture to commit to that process of discovery?

In the Occupy Wall Street movement that began in the autumn of 2011, people came together in Zuccotti Park in Manhattan to protest the immoral activities of large banking institutions. After the protest had gone on for a while, seasoned activists saw the population of these protests was quite different from the norm. People who had recently lost their homes due to illegal mortgage deals and college students and people who had been living on the street for years gathered together and camped out in the public park for weeks. The movement quickly spread to roughly 1400 cities, all over the world. People who were not the 1% of the population, considered the wealthy elite of the world, began to identify as the other 99% and the alchemical process began. Barbara Ehrenreich gives her journalist's perspective on this movement:

Here were thousands of people—we may never know the exact numbers—from all walks of life, living outdoors in the streets and parks, very much as the poorest of the poor have always lived: without electricity, heat, water, or toilets. In the process, they managed to create self-governing communities. General assembly meetings brought together an unprecedented mix of recent college graduates, young professionals, elderly people, laid-off blue-collar workers, and plenty of the chronically homeless for what were, for the most part, constructive and civil exchanges. What started as a diffuse protest against economic injustice became a vast experiment in class building...In fact, the encampments engendered almost unthinkable convergences: people from comfortable backgrounds learning about street survival from the homeless, a distinguished professor of political science discussing horizontal versus vertical decision-making with a postal worker...."[4]

When it was announced that the police would remove the Occupy Portland encampment by midnight on November 12, 2011, I felt concerned that police might become violent if the protestors used nonviolent resistance. I have noticed that public support, actual bodies, and cameras really change the mood of those kinds of situations. Supposedly, in the US, we have the right to protest, to make free speech and people deserve to do these things without being beaten or hurt. I decided to go to the encampment, along with a few friends, to see what we could do to change the energy, witness the process, support peaceful behavior from all parties.

The encampment was scheduled to be removed at midnight if the protestors did not disperse. We arrived at quarter to midnight, carrying candles and handmade signs and just stared at the scene, struck wordless. The streets were filled with thousands of people to support the Occupiers and the police chose not to disperse the encampment at that time. People remained in the streets, dancing and drumming and singing until early the next morning. Protestors marched in the streets of downtown Portland carrying supportive signs and riding bikes around the encampment.

All of the encampments were eventually broken up but something did ignite and transformation began. A sense of solidarity had sprung up, even among very unlikely companions to create public opposition to the economic realities people were facing. Even people not involved in the encampments moved their money out of the large banks that were practicing unethical methods for their mortgages. The Occupy movement took many people's painful stories about money and loss and created a platform for connection and social change. As a result, neighbors created support and resistance for families who were in danger of losing their homes to the banks. US politicians are addressing financial concerns in a more candid way than has happened in the past. There is no knowing what this alchemical experiment will uncover but it served as a wake-up call to an otherwise jaded and overwhelmed nation.

There is a pattern that you tell yourself has held you back more than anything. It's time to begin to ask it what its job is. Why did it come to you? When did it form? What purpose did it have in the beginning? What protection has it offered during your life? "That's just the way it is" isn't going to cut it anymore. How can we begin to take the first step towards alchemical transformation? We see the cracks, we see the possibility. We can put one hand on each side of it and peel it open, wash it, transform it utterly into the strength that it has always wanted to be. Alchemy tells us that we cannot dismiss the wound. Our wounds offer us inspiration, tell us what matters to us, and often point us in the direction of our life's healing work. Nothing is more courageous than to take a holy risk and take your place as a wounded healer.

Revolutionary Healing Dares:

I dare you to list the most tender and difficult pieces of your past on paper or aloud. I dare you to hold them gently and consider taking them through the fire, the water, the air, and the earth to see what spiritual gold lies within. I dare you to be audacious in the transformations you dream of and ask for. The first step is often the most difficult and the most crucial.

I dare you to take it. I dare you to hold the stories of other people with the utmost respect and offer them the hope that something that they have survived or are currently enduring will become their most valuable jewel. I dare you to help the people whose lives you touch find magnificence in their metamorphoses.

Spiritual Inventory:
Exercises for Alchemy

1. **Journal writing:** What is the story about your health or illness that holds you back? What would you change about yourself if you had a magic wand? What is the primary issue that is not serving you in your life right now? What would have to transform in your life for this to shift?

2. **The Wounded Healer:** Claim your wounds and gifts:

   What is your greatest gift or skill? When do you remember using it or having it acknowledged?

   What was the hardest thing about your childhood? When did it begin? What developed as a result? When do you use these resulting skills in your life, job, and relationships today?

   Write or draw about these wounds and gifts. Imagine holding one in one hand and one in the other. Pour two cups of water half full and call one Wounds and the other, Gifts. Play with pouring them into each other, making an imaginary alchemical formula of your Wounded Healer qualities.

3. **Human Resources Director:** Remember your reactive state personality from Chapter 7. What would it be like to change your relationship with that part of you and reassign them to a new job? What else could this part of you do other than defend you? Write the old job that this reactive personality used to fulfill on a sheet of non-bleached paper. Then, literally add the elements of water, fire, earth, air to the page and change it completely. You can take the ashes or sludge or mud and bury it or add it to the soil of a house plant or use it in clay to create something new. Use your global revolutionary healer imagination.

   Next, write this part of yourself a letter to inform them of their promotion. For instance, a strong flight/escape response could be put in charge of planning vacations. Find a way to remind yourself of the change the next time this old pattern wants to come up and ask it to do the new job instead.

Living Inspiration: Lorie Dechar

Lorie Dechar is a visionary acupuncturist, psychologist, alchemist, mentor, and teacher, who lives in Downeast Maine. She is the author of *Five Spirits: Alchemical Acupuncture for Psychological and Spiritual Healing*, a guide to the Five Spirits of Chinese medicine and Taoist psycho-spiritual alchemy. I participated in her yearlong mentorship to explore alchemy in a contemporary context and found her expertise in the treatment room and classroom to be outstanding. We discussed alchemy in our times.

LD: I'm so glad you are writing this book now. We are in a paradigm shift. Our predominant culture may be disintegrating but it is still ruled by rational patriarchal consciousness. The dualism of this currently dominant consciousness separates the cosmos and our being into parts. It emphatically favors what Taoist alchemists considered the Yang upper spirits. These upper spirits relate to aspects of our psyche associated with conscious thought, the mind, and heaven. From the perspective of this dualistic consciousness, the lower spirits that are associated with the body and instincts, with our ancestral wisdom, embodied knowing, and the earth are viewed as shadow. As shadow, the lower spirits are less valued and are often maligned as dangerous and demonic. While this is still the culture in which we live, the dominant paradigm is beginning to shift. This is a big part of the Revolution of the Spirit that you are speaking about. It is the shift we are just beginning to see in medicine and other significant areas of our culture.

I want to clarify that I don't see the work of integrating the shadow as separate from any of the work we are called to do as contemporary alchemists. I'm getting clear that the whole realm of the lower spirits—the realm of our unconscious bodily impulses and the wisdom of the collective unconscious—is typically left out of mainstream conversations, in particular the discourse of traditional behavioral therapies, coaching, counseling, and psycho-pharmacology. In these current psychological approaches, there is often an idea that to reach a goal, we can set an intention and move toward it with a plan that we follow step-by-step. We leave no room for the chaos and unpredictable energy that comes from below. To embrace this uncertainty opens us to a radically different attitude that confronts many of the kinds of therapies currently being practiced.

GRS: Yes, the extreme nature of our orientation toward a goal is hard to navigate. Hopefully to reengage with alchemy is a more inclusive attitude that could lead to more holistic success, maybe not immediately, but over time.

LD: Success may look very different than we think it should. We can have goals and objectives but we have to make room for all that we don't know and how our goals might change over time, with life events, with further information.

GRS: Where do you personally see a hunger for the sacred the most?

LD: Where I see that hunger the most is in every aspect of life that has to do with the lower spirits, particularly the parts of our lives that come under the jurisdiction of what the ancient Taoists called the Po soul and the Zhi spirit.

In very short hand, the Po is the animating life force of the autonomic nervous system, of our human instinctual nature, our gut longings and body responses that may be unconscious but are still central to our being. When the Po soul is ignored, the body's innate wisdom is lost. That is where I see the most emptiness, the greatest hunger for the sacred. When the voice of the body is silenced, the sacredness of the lower spirits, the body and matter are pushed into the shadow. In response to this repression, a vast array of symptoms arise including depression, self-destructive habits, accumulation of belongings we don't need, chronic pain, and loneliness to mention just a few of the most common ones we see regularly in the treatment room.

In the Taoist alchemy texts, the Zhi spirit is the animating life force of our inherited instinctual nature. It is the most high-grade energy of the body. The Zhi regulates more than just our personal nervous system. The Zhi spirit is the carrier of our ancestral traits, the wisdom that comes to us through our bloodline and our DNA. It is our very will to survive and carry on our genetic inheritance but beyond this, the Zhi endows us with the capacity to truly surrender to the divine. The Zhi connects us to the collective unconscious, the part of the psyche that draws us out from and back into the infinite. It is related to the power of the life force, cosmic will, and the driving urgency of ambition. When this aspect of our being is not honored, we see symptoms such as adrenal burnout, insomnia, sexual addiction, fertility issues, degenerative bone and spine disorders, again just to mention a few of the symptoms often seen in modern Western patients.

I see the hunger for the sacred right now in people's attitude toward money. People think that they want more and more and yet, unconsciously ask, "Can I gain enough quantity of stuff to make me feel okay?" There is an insatiable hunger for security, money, clothes, food, relationships, sex that comes when spirit is absent from a human life. This lack of spirit is a disaster for us on personal as well as planetary levels. It is the true epidemic of our time. If the lower spirits—the Po or Zhi—are maligned or repressed, there is a voracious appetite; an accumulating of "stuff" in a futile attempt to satisfy our longing for our own embodied spirituality. A person whose life is devoid of spirit may have many material belongings but there will be no quality of life, no meaning, and no depth.

GRS: How did alchemy come to be a vital part of your life and work? Why is it of value to you?

LD: Years ago, in the midst of my own personal journey, I felt as if my life was falling apart. I left my daughter's father and was feeling depressed, alone, and very frightened. I was uncertain of my course and wasn't even sure I wanted to practice acupuncture anymore. I had never felt anything like this before and I was desperately trying to heal and put my life back together. I moved from doing acupuncture to exploring Western psychology. I started by studying Gestalt and Focusing and although I still use techniques drawn from these types of therapy, I did not feel that they were able to answer my deepest questions. I had not yet found a way to heal myself or to integrate Western and Taoist attitudes toward psycho-spiritual healing. When I discovered Archetypal Psychology and Jung's work with alchemy, I realized that I had found the integrating factor. Alchemical principles are at the core of Chinese medicine as well as Jung's work. Alchemy gives us a language with which we can talk about the soul. Through alchemy, I found a healing modality that could help me go through the challenges of true psycho-spiritual healing and transformation.

This kind of transformation is not just changing or tweaking behavior or understanding why you keep doing something that isn't working. Real transformation means letting structures come apart so something new can form. While this understanding was personally valuable in my own healing process, it also gave me a way to reframe what is happening on a planetary level as our human consciousness goes through disintegrations and reorganization. There is a collective movement of healing happening right now. Through the lens of alchemy, we can begin to see the uncertainty and chaos of our world as not just a frightening event but as a necessary part of transformational processes, a process of gestation rather than a problem to fix.

When I started to get this, it helped me understand the impasse that had happened at the close of the revolution of the sixties when so many visionary changes had begun but somehow never fully manifested on a cultural level. I was in high school during the '60s and the flower children movement influenced the way that I was learning to look at the world. But the skills and strengths needed to come apart and reform, a sense of how to maneuver through the powerful transits of deep change, these require a kind of seasoned maturity, a willingness to bear suffering. During that first round of cultural change, the first round of this revolution of the spirit that took place in the '60s, there was a lot of light but no way to move through darkness. Shamans in other cultures were probably skilled at moving through these chaos states but we collectively didn't have those skills. One of the reasons why I like to listen to young people who are coming of age now is that they are starting to formulate new ways of navigating descent processes and chaos. I see that some of these ideas are beginning to mature in these times.

GRS: And when we find new ways of being in our descent, we can integrate some of the cultural pieces that are in the shadows.

LD: Interesting that you say that because in alchemy, the integration always happens in the *nigredo*, the shadow or darkening that is the night-sea journey of the soul.

GRS: Why is the concept of alchemy important to our collective health?

LD: Alchemy complements our modern rational worldview. It fills in the blanks of modern science. It gives us a language and a way of organizing experience that brings soul back into the world of matter. While modern science quantifies the world, alchemy deals with qualities of experience. While modern science analyzes and takes things apart, alchemy integrates, relates, and weaves the world back into wholeness. As a collective, it's crucial for us to find a way to reconnect quantity and quality, matter and spirit. We need to find a way to reconnect with the nonquantifiable, ineffable aspects of life, to be able to go to the depths of our own being and find ways to tolerate uncertainty, constraint, suffering, and disintegration. We need to root our spiritual longings in the rich soil of our bodies and our lives. Alchemy offers us the tools we need in order to work and heal at these very deep levels of being.

GRS: Yes, we certainly turn away from chaos and our own depths as a culture and consider this realm as distasteful and undesirable. It makes it very lonely if you are the one in that uncertain state of being.

LD: The alchemists recognized these states as essential to transformation. They used the model of the five elements or the cycle of birth, growth, death, disintegration, and renewal. This view is used in all the alchemical traditions.

GRS: It's also visible in the natural world.

LD: Yes, it is the way of nature, the way of the embodied spirit. If we resist this cycle of change, we get stuck, sick, depressed, and stunted. If we cannot die, we cannot be reborn. Ultimately, our spirit loses its brightness if it is not reinvigorated through the process of descent.

GRS: This is important to us personally but perhaps also builds capacity for us to engage with each other on a cultural level.

LD: Right now, when someone dies, it is often considered a failure in medicine. Death, from the perspective of modern Western culture and Western medicine, is the ultimate shadow because we don't hold it as a sacred archetype. As long as the health care system makes death the enemy rather than a crucial part of the life cycle and the healing process, there is no way to come to a place of collective health. We are stuck in an endless loop in which there is no way out.

GRS: I'm interested in provocation around these things; what are we afraid would happen if we included death in our experience of health?

LD: There is no way that we can solve the problem with health care for the culture unless we radically change our attitude toward death, the unknown, the processes of disintegration, and the relinquishing of personal will. To the ancient Taoists, the Dark Goddess, Xi Wang Mu, Queen Mother of the West ruled this aspect of the life cycle. Although the Dark Goddess was feared, she was also honored as the guardian of the doorways of life and death and the progenitor of transformation, rebirth, and new possibilities.

GRS: What are the side effects of a world where people don't honor this part of life and don't value alchemical transformation? What do you see as the major barriers to including these practices in the world we live in?

LD: One of the side effects is that people desperately resist change. There is no spiritual or cultural support for people who need to surrender to transformation. Sometimes that transformation means physical death but often in a healing process, it is really about letting go of an old way of being, letting go of outmoded or self-destructive thought or behavior patterns or letting a part of our identity die. This kind of surrender is incredibly difficult. It is a spiritual vision quest that requires courage and fortitude as well as a committed and seasoned guide. Our current health care system has almost no way to support us in doing it. Instead, we focus on fixing the body in the same way we fix a machine. We focus on "getting back to our old self again" instead of discovering new possibilities. But this attitude does not make sense, even from a rational point of view. It is "the old self" that got us sick in the first place and the human body is much more than its machinery. Without valuing the soul and the necessity of transformational processes, we get stuck in endless, repetitive cycles and are unable to move on, to grow, to transform psychologically and spiritually. There is no way out within the existing paradigm. We have to rediscover our relationship to the Dark Goddess archetype, the ultimate power and divinity of the Earth and of biological processes. The major barrier is still, unfortunately, patriarchy.

GRS: That brings us back to our unconscious heritage of Puritanism, colonialism, and dualism.

LD: Yes, as a culture, with our Puritanical heritage, we still have a definite preference for the Yang and a clear bias toward the upper spirits—the light, bright, clear, and active aspects of psychic energy. Our negative attitude toward the Yin, the dark, subtle, receptive, and gestational aspects of our being is still a barrier to wholeness, planetary healing, and new possibilities for consciousness. It becomes more and more painful, an almost cellular suffering, as we want to change but we don't know how. By making the possibilities and wisdom of alchemy known, we have more options.

GRS: What do you think would change in the world if alchemy became integrated in our culture or available within our systems of medicine? For instance, what would be altered if people could choose to code surviving cancer as a kind of alchemical transformation process?

LD: When alchemical principles and tools are integrated into healing, people's unique, personal experiences become part of the process. We no longer leave our body knowing, our dreams, our addictions, our quirks, and our passions at the door of the treatment room. Pain and suffering—depression, digestive disturbances, chronic pain, anxiety, even cancer—are no longer simply problems to be fixed but rather opportunities for psycho-spiritual transformation and growth. Our symptoms point us in the direction of new possibilities. From an alchemical perspective, we don't just focus on making symptoms go away, but rather we want to glean their meaning. We want to discover how our suffering can help us move forward. In this way, we leave behind the idea of the quick fix as the only success. Instead, alchemy seeks to discover how our lead can become our gold.

GRS: What is your offering to these interesting times in terms of your work? What does the world need most right now in order to return to healthy culture?

LD: My unique contribution begins with my commitment to understanding, harnessing, and teaching the alchemical underpinnings of Traditional Chinese Medicine. I think I have brought forth a new appreciation and cherishing of the lower spirits and supported the creation of practices that help people as they descend into the lower realms—the irrational, instinctual, and emotional realms of the Yin, the body and the embodied soul. These lower realms are often very unfamiliar and frightening to those of us who have grown up in a dualistic culture that values the rational mind and the disembodied spirit and yet they are the only place where real transformation can actually occur. Another area where I have sought to make a contribution is in supporting the shift from the currently predominant rational, linear, dualistic consciousness to a more multidimensional, holistic, integral awareness. A hallmark of this new consciousness is that it recognizes the divinity that is immanent and palpably present in the material world. Obviously, this is a fundamental necessity if we are to bring spirit back to medicine and radically renew our ideas about the healing process. To this end, I have created advanced training programs for practitioners who want to move beyond the limitations of our current consciousness structure, who are committed to bringing soul and spirit back to the realm of healing. My goal and greatest hope is to support each person I work with in discovering their individual divinity and how this divinity can manifest in their life and in their world. All my tools are in service of individuals finding their own unique magic. That is where we need to go as a culture. Each of us has to find that light and knowing inside. That creates a culture of empowered, enlivened humans.

GRS: Some of the most interesting unknowns are about what happens when we come alive as individuals and start to come together collaboratively to change our relationships to spirit, to each other, and to the planet. How do you see this happening?

LD: The Cultural Revolution took place in China from 1966–1976. During this time, a new level of materialism was imposed on the Chinese people. There was an irrevocable split between spirit and matter and any reference to spiritual practices in healing or elsewhere were violently suppressed. The early Western radicals who brought Chinese medicine to the West in the mid-1970s were also coming from a Marxist perspective. Like the Chinese communists, they did not value the spirituality of Chinese medicine but were looking for an alternative medicine that could be made widely available to people who had little or no access to mainstream Western medicine. They imported Mao Zedong's version of Chinese medicine. This modernized style of acupuncture and herbal medicine was formulaic, materialistic, and intentionally devoid of psychological concern or any reference to spirituality.

My teacher, J. R. Worsley, didn't go in that direction. He tried to bring his own view of spirituality to the teaching and practice of Chinese medicine and that is why I gravitated to his style of acupuncture. Through my 27 years of practice, I have continued to search for ways to bring soul and spirit into my treatment room.

Now that China's Cultural Revolution is well behind us and many patients are actively looking for more holistic ways to heal, it is that much more upsetting to me that Taoist and alchemical spiritual principles and practices are still largely ignored in the teaching of this medicine. Of course, leaving the mysterious "spiritual parts" out makes it much easier to integrate Chinese medicine into Western clinical settings, to fill out insurance forms, and to develop licensing regulations and standardized testing, but to me, it is a betrayal of this ancient tradition as well as of its students, practitioners, and patients. Many schools have not yet taken on what it would mean to actually teach from a radically different paradigm. Because of this, the most profound impact Chinese medicine could have in the transformation of modern Western culture and consciousness is still not happening.

GRS: Or the spirituality of the medicine is mentioned here and there in schools but it is not being lived or practiced.

LD: Yes, it is a matter of living, being, and practicing differently rather than just paying lip service to an idea of including spirit in our healing work. It is about being willing to suffer the dismemberments of divine energies as they penetrate and reorganize the structures of our lives. So I am going to keep writing, teaching, and voicing the work of the original alchemists and I am gratified to know that, despite the challenges and opposition, there are other people deeply committed to this kind of alchemical healing. There is a potent stream coming through to us from the original Taoist alchemical texts that is a living treasure but it is important to recognize that this is not just more information that can be lightly taught and quickly learned. This alchemical wisdom comes up from down below. It must be felt and lived in order to be understood. In this way, it is revolutionary! And it is wonderfully subversive, a threat to the dominant paradigm.

GRS: Then and now, why is it such a threat?

LD: Alchemy boggles the rational mind and undermines top-down forms of authority and knowledge. It values individual experience, chaos, confusion, and the potency of the imagination. It honors the wisdom of organic processes. It recognizes the divine in the light of heaven but also in the moist, fertile darkness of the earth. We who are working with this stuff have a common language about it that has to be shared. We have to find our way back to honoring the living archetype of the Dark Goddess, her voice and the resonance of her terrain.

GRS: I was recently reading about the author imprisoned during the Maoist Revolution for teaching the I Ching; what is so threatening about studying a spiritual map for change?

LD: Even as Chinese medicine is more and more accepted, there is a fundamental misunderstanding about what the Taoist alchemists believed. Many teachers still focus on the transcendence of matter and the body as the ultimate goal of our spiritual practices. All too often, we hear texts interpreted to mean that the upper spirits must rule over the lower. But on the most fundamental level, if we look more carefully at the texts and etymology of the earliest Chinese characters, we find that the alchemical wisdom texts—including ancient Taoist alchemical texts, early medical texts, as well as the I Ching—posit a view of the world where Yin and Yang, masculine and feminine, spirit and matter, mind and body, above and below are equal partners in the cosmic dance. Yang ultimately does not hold ascendency or power over Yin. Neither does Yin dominate Yang. Rather the two emerge simultaneously from the swirling infinite potentiality of Tao—the unknowable creative matrix of the universe. Yin and Yang create and destroy each other in the endless multidimensional hologram of life. As healers and visionaries, we must stand for the equality and essential integrity of the upper and lower spirits. We must view descent as an equal partner to ascent in transformational processes. The necessity of this revisioning cannot be overstated. The real revolution here is our commitment to holding the lower spirits of earth, body, and matter as equal in value to the upper spirits of heaven and the mind.

GRS: I keep coming back to the fact that the personal and cultural situation we are in is not an intellectual problem, rather it's experiential and the solutions must be passed through teaching and living.

LD: Yes, we keep creating the world through the words we speak, the practices we embody, the visions we manifest, and the relationships we nurture and cherish. Most of all, it is through our capacity to know, see, speak, love, and be in the world differently that the world will change. To me, this is the essence of true healing.

CHAPTER TEN

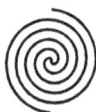

Initiation: The Journey Across The Threshold

You can wish for something
fevered,
sweating.
You can pray for something
on your knees,
forehead pressed to the floor.
But
if you mean it,
you will conjure
something from nothing.
A song from brutal silence,
unfolds hidden wings.
Your patience
is a whispered syllable
of the secret name of your heart
into the ear of some wild god
with a water gift.
The difference between a prayer
and a spell
is audacity.

The difference between restoration
and transformation
is a cocoon.
The difference between your comfort
and your journey
is surrender
and sometimes resistance.
When you know the difference,
you are free.

– GRS

∞

At age 23, I am seeking a rite of passage to celebrate my adult-
hood and to search for answers about my career path. I go on a
vision quest in southwestern New Mexico with an experienced
guide who facilitates four days of solo camping, fasting, praying, and
witnessing. He translates the vision quest experience from the way that
indigenous people used it to contemporary times, noting the lack of ritual in our modern urban culture. The first day is lovely, still and not
incredibly hard. The second day is lonely and I find it difficult to con-
centrate because of the hunger. I keep daydreaming about chocolate,
avocados, cheese, seafood, apples, fantasizing about the meals I will eat
when this is done. It was suggested that we perform a symbolic death
ritual on the second day, imagining ourselves giving thanks and saying
goodbye to the people and experiences in our lives. I do a ritual like this,
naming all of the people I have met and loved and lost and how they
have touched me. I break down crying about how amazing my life is,
how grateful I am to have experienced both the beautiful and hurtful
times, how sad I am that I have taken so much for granted. On the third
day of no food and only drinking water from a nearby spring, I wake up
feeling slightly lightheaded but very clear. I climb out of my sleeping bag
and watch the earth itself rise and fall with a rhythmic breath. It does
not stop when I close my eyes and reopen them. Each tree appears to
be engaging in this rhythm, moving ever so slightly as the earth inhales
and exhales.

A 45 year-old patient comes to me after being newly diagnosed with breast cancer. She talks about her first chemotherapy appointment and how she is not sure that she wants to complete her course of chemo. "The chemo is making me sicker than the cancer, but I fear that if I stop, I will die and leave my children alone." She talks about how alone she feels at work, people are sympathetic but don't really know what to say to her. She feels separate, alien, and angry. I talk briefly about death/rebirth initiations in other cultures and ask if anything about that feels similar to her experience. She nods emphatically, "That is exactly what is happening. I feel like I'm getting initiated and I have no idea what I will be like after this or what's going to happen to me. It's terrifying."

Sacred Exploration:

Initiation is one way of coding arduous or painful experiences as death/rebirth journeys, a view of a big change with a transformational lens. Seeing a life transition as an initiatory crossing can become a vital perspective on change and suffering, to give it a wider purpose. This is something that humans have traditionally done to help each other hold a "big picture" and pass wisdom from the more experienced to the less experienced members of community. Thomas Berry, a Catholic monk and universal philosopher, says "One of the most frequent archetypes is the performance of death and rebirth ceremonies. Humans are not fully human until they've gone through some ceremonial rebirth."

A traditional initiation in an indigenous culture would likely begin with a symbolic death and culminate in a rebirth ritual. In many cultures, young people would be initiated in small groups, generally organized by gender. Their rite of passage from child to adult permitted them to become fully functioning members of the tribe. How then does the use of initiation as a model affect our human health and spiritual development in contemporary times?

It is said that the only thing we can count on is change. However, when changes come, we can feel inundated and alienated from our families and communities. We know that life changes are normal and many are inevitable. People die, work changes, relationships end. This isn't new information. We are fully aware that shift will happen. It is still impossible to prepare for the effect of these transitions on our lives. I am regularly amazed at how much of my life force energy I spend guarding against the unavoidable changes that are coming, rather than savoring every exquisite moment of my days. I will never be ready for my life to alter itself in the striking ways that it does. I have absolutely no control over this.

The context of initiation is valuable because life always holds the inevitability of potentially devastating experiences. Our ability to change our perception helps us to survive the most difficult situations. Initiation is very much an alchemical process.

Using the model of a death-rebirth cycle to code our struggles gives us some sense of hopefulness that may otherwise feel far away. Remembering that time is not only linear can remind us to seek the possibility of rebirth even in the midst of pain. In this archetypal pattern, death is not the end. Rebirth always pursues it. Other people have made it through this. You will not always feel this way. The trying times right now will not last forever. You are never alone.

Initiation offers a toolbox for those of us experiencing suffering. Often, what is the most difficult about a life change is the passing of the way it was before the difference happened. The second most difficult part is the acceptance of the unfamiliar reality and attempt to create life anew. We rarely have any jurisdiction over the modifications that life makes; we can only determine our reply to them. What have people before us done to move through these situations? How might we transform our present sense of hurt into future wisdom?

David Richo, a psychotherapist, educator and author, reminds us that "it is precisely the pain and shock of the initiation ceremony that initiates...we are always dying to what is not essential."[1] We can either shrink from the aspects of our life cycles that feel like death or we can recognize them as a crucial part of the process. We do not have any significant incentive to release our comfort or the parts of our stories that are already known. Initiation can give us inspiration to more gracefully release our illusions of control and move into the mystery. Seeing our life events through the eyes of a candidate facing initiation firmly removes us from our self-deceptions of victimization and invites us back to empowerment.

As a global revolutionary healer, you have passed through something to get where you are. No healer becomes a healer without an initiation of some sort. There are the kind of initiations that we choose to go through formally with mentors and challenges that we can understand. There are also the kinds of initiations that choose us and we often don't understand what is happening until we are deep within it, or possibly on the other side. You may be in the midst of an initiation right now. There are simple parts to it and sometimes they even happen in order.

In modern times, there are few opportunities for the formal pursuit of initiation for people who do not seek to become healers, teachers or spiritual leaders. But the process of initiation is still a vital paradigm from which we can draw courage. What usually happens first is that life deviates from the everyday reality. This can be a cataclysm or a gradual uneasiness that something is different. The initiate is set upon the path. Sometimes that path leads down into an 'underworld' realm in many stories from around the world. There is often an unwanted or unplanned period of shedding, cleansing or loss.

Most initiations are characterized by the endurance or completion of challenges Sometimes these challenges are physical, designed to prove commitment to the process. Many people describe their experience of a recovery from an illness to be an initiatory experience. If they heal, they emerge with a greater fidelity to their lives and dedication to their health. Sometimes the challenges are mental/emotional or spiritual; the candidate must complete tasks, face some inner demons, learn a practice, or devote to something.

Candidates for initiation are often asked to pass a test or exhibit bravery in a dangerous situation, whether the danger is real or perceived, before coming to the initiation ceremony itself. In many indigenous cultures, initiation asks that something precious to the candidate be released in order to create an opening for the rebirth experience. In initiation ceremonies, the candidate will often have to pass over some kind of a threshold. The successful crossing of this threshold is often the key to the beginning of the ritual. There are challengers or guardians waiting at this gate who ask the candidate a question or pose a threat that must be overcome. The symbolic death or sacrifice is necessary to reveal the circumstances for impending birth. Passing through that gate can be excruciating but when it's done, you trust your ability to make it even through the most intense initiations. You will not be the same.

Another characteristic of many initiations is that there are mysteries or core truths that are passed to the person after crossing the threshold, completing the challenges and participating in the ritual. Our perseverance is rewarded and we receive wisdom from a source beyond ourselves. These might not even be lessons that are conveyed in words nor understood solely with the intellect. These gifts are integrated somehow into the initiate's being before celebrating the individual's progress, journey, and arrival at the other side or return home.

After initiation, the person who has passed over the threshold carries more experience, power and a newfound sense of self. You will know more about what your soul wants to experience and communicate when you have reached the other side. These initiations are often a place to begin to speak, write or sing from. You will be even more yourself.

Sometimes there is a new name that the initiate takes, or a new title/role in community. There is also a greater degree of insight after initiation and the acknowledgment of a clear initiator who led the way, whether that be another person or the experience itself. The gifts of initiation, along with a sense of accomplishment and wisdom, can include the duty to hold the container for others in the same process. There is some kind of leadership or service that is expected, or at least role modeling from someone who has been through this experience.

What can service mean in these contemporary times? In modern times, the intensity of our life stress and personal problems may obscure any obligation to those outside of our immediate family or friendship circle. In the absence of tribe, we search for communities who hold values that are similar to ours. It is a human need to feel useful, to believe that one's life experiences have meaning that goes beyond the personal. There are so many places and people who need help in our own towns and in our world. Where can we be the most effective?

To whom are we responsible?

An initiation can be a highly individualized experience, but the completion of it will often carry a commitment to aid or teach others. Survivors of an illness are often asked to share their stories with folks who have recently been diagnosed. The twelve step recovery community uses a system where an individual who has been working the program longer sponsors someone who is newly sober. Those who live through childhood abuse and find peace and function in their lives provide needed models to others who don't believe it possible. When we are suffering, we are hungry for details of what to expect, hungry for examples that we hold when we feel we can't go on. It is a service to tell these stories of our own deaths and rebirths and give people hope that they too can survive and thrive. People want to hear about what you have understood in your struggles. I promise.

The completion of an initiation can ignite the call to service within us, highlighting our passions and showing us that without which our lives would not be worthwhile. People who have been through a traumatic experience often say that afterward, they stop taking their life for granted, that they somehow wake up and begin to appreciate more subtle things. Perhaps, initiation allows us to remove many layers of distraction from our lives or dissolve some of the compartmentalization that keeps us separate from the world around us.

What initiations have you experienced? Were they mindful excursions or sudden explosions? Who helped you cross the threshold or lit the dark way for you? For whom are you acting as initiator, consciously or not? How could you be of service to others who are stepping onto this path? Even as wounded healers, we hold the lantern and offer assistance to others wandering in the darkness.

Revolutionary Healing Dares:

I dare you to acknowledge the initiations that you have passed through in order to stand here today. I dare you to make a list of them from the present day all the way back to your birth and read it out loud to yourself. I dare you to notice whether or not you are involved in an initiation process right now and ask yourself who can guide you to the doorway. I dare you to take stock of what responsibility you might take based on what you have learned through your own adventure through the gates. I dare you to act in joyful service to another, asking them what they need to cross their threshold and trusting yourself to know what is helpful based on your own journey. I urge you to discover where you can be of service to the life force and animating spirit in all things.

Spiritual Inventory: Exercises for Initiation

1. **Journal:** Are you in an initiation now? Have you finished one and are trying to integrate it? What have you lost? What is shifting dramatically? What are your challenges? What new possibility is coming into being? How have you changed?

2. **Celebration:** Throw a party or cook a dinner to celebrate your changes. You can invite others if you want or make it a ritual

feast for yourself. Write a toast describing where you have been and where you have arrived and/or invite others to make their own toasts acknowledging changes and transformations that they have made in their lives.

3. **Service:** Determine if there are people known to you who are going through a similarly difficult time to what you have survived. How can you help them? Can you write to them, listen to them, volunteer, offer advice, give a talk, or donate money?

Living Inspiration: Robert Birch

Robert Birch is an activist, educator, and longtime advocate for gay rights and people who are living with HIV. He has created trainings, academic work, and art around the concept of illness as a rite of passage. He lives on Salt Spring Island in British Columbia and teaches internationally. We talked about using the archetypal pattern of initiation as a lens through which to view illness or crisis.

GRS: Where do you personally see a hunger for the sacred the most?

RB: I see it in our desire to connect. It is essential to our well-being. However habitual or unconscious our actions are, much of what we do is an attempt toward or a denial of connection. When we embrace intimacy, we are embraced by the sacred. We become erotically engaged, more fully aware of the cycles of life and our sense of place.

What inhibits intimacy? Hegemonic culture acts as a deterrent to true desire, destabilizing a livelier sense of self-in-community. Mainstream culture opposes health. It desensitizes our instincts, has us feeding off dead ideas and empty foods, and numbs us out to its gladiator culture of violence and fear.

The work I do gently examines how illness resensitizes us. Illness is often ruthless, it insists we change or be changed. Whether as host or caregiver, illness reawakens us to what's immediate. Pain demands attention. From the perspective of archetypal psychology, it propels us into the underworld. It seems our body and our world betrayed us. Personal illusions and expectations get stripped away. Illness is an agent of change; it casts us into a healing crisis. Illness embodies soul. It thrusts us into a sacred drama. Serious illness casts us as a peon in an ageless struggle between Thanatos and Eros, where the gods of death and life strive for supremacy. The body becomes the dramatic stage where this mythic battle erupts. The impossible is asked of us. At one's most depleted the heroic is demanded. In despair, we enter a dark night of the soul.

As with most shocks, initially we bargain, we plea, rage, grieve, and eventually surrender. We then learn to ask for help. Ideally, this brings us back into relationships rooted in appreciation. We are more vulnerable and tender together. Our world begins to expand out of necessity. At this time core values and purpose can also reemerge. "I want to get better! I cannot do it alone." We connect.

Cultures more rooted in the natural world understood that biology and beliefs are interwoven. Beyond some new age concept, healing is a rebirth, often painful, potentially glorious, the return to the spark of life. This spark exists as a communion: in community, in nature, in creativity.

Healing is more than getting better. Healing is a profound act of transformation. Deep healing is its own revolution: biological, perceptional, soulful, and cultural. It is a return to the erotic. The erotic has the ability to further detoxify us from that which has previously been deadened within us. Illness has the potential to assist our psyches to confront and surrender up what has not been life-inducing. Illness directs our attention back to our primary desires, the need for touch, to know health as freedom, to play in and connect to nature, to know ourselves *as* nature. Whatever the outcome of the process, be it health or death, by giving our full attention to our erotic nature we have the potential to revitalize some of what matters most to us.

GRS: Terry Tempest Williams says, "Erotic is what those deep relationships are and can be that engage the whole body—our heart, our mind, our spirit, our flesh. It is that moment of being exquisitely present."

RB: Yes, present moment awareness, intimacy. Sacredness calls us to what we are hungry for—meaning, belonging, and purpose. The erotic, and paradoxically, illness, ignites all three of these functions. I often think of the improbable tension of paradox. How is illness in and of itself healing? How is the death journey a summons to the erotic? How do we make sickness an expression of the sacred? To sacrifice is to make sacred. What does illness ask us to sacrifice so we might feel connected? Deep healing requires imagination.

The sacred shows up in these feelings of timelessness, when we feel richly connected, momentarily touched by the unseen world.

GRS: Do you feel we have access to timelessness in everyday life?

RB: From leisurely strolls with friends to accidents and unexpected events, yes we do, but it's not inherently present in our turbulent culture. Active engagement with creativity, sensuality, nature, travel, meditation, forms of intimacy and/or ecstasy can awaken this sense of time out of time. Because time is consensus-based, anything that interrupts this social construct has the potential to be sacred. It is healing when we experience timelessness as a conscious process rather than a reactive one.

Initiation is also a path to connect with the sacred. Understanding crisis as an unexpected opening to a new world brings us to the threshold of initiation and therefore the sacred. Crisis perceived as initiatory concerns both personal and collective processes of change.

Feminist principle has taught us that the personal is political. We are also an expression of the generational and historical. In personal initiation it could be said that we are doing the work of ourselves and our ancestors simultaneously. By embracing this concept we promote agency rather than pathology. Today's health care system is built on foundations of individual behavioral pathology, which only leads to further disassociation, victimization, and trauma. Beyond any romantic view of violence or trauma, we have always needed one another to learn how to heal through suffering, how to face terror with courage and resiliency. To truly find one another through the labyrinth of our pain is a sacred journey. At times harrowing, this task is an archetypal journey. Not only our sovereignty is at risk, but the health and wellness of family and societal systems.

GRS: How did the archetype of initiation come to be a vital part of your life and work? Why is it of value to you?

RB: The notion of illness as a rite of passage came to me initially through two events. The first was a diagnosis of HIV at age twenty-seven, then during a two-year period as the primary caregiver for my husband's encounter with AIDS. In both cases, I was not in an urban epicenter of AIDS so the trauma was initially personal. I had to rely on the internal skills I had and the love of my friends and family. I remember instinctively rebelling against the term "HIV positive" and so renamed it for myself as, "I host HIV." Or defiantly, arrogantly said to myself, "I am not this virus, I *live* with HIV and, live or die, HIV will transform my life. It will teach me what I need to learn." I then fell into a three month state of depression, my initial descent into the underworld.

I both embraced and resisted responsibility for the diagnosis. Personal actions are part of a larger cultural paradigm of privilege and social oppression. All illness is extremely personal and simultaneously bigger than any individual. Like many gay men, because of HIV, I had to come out all over again. This impacted my family; it asked them to confront issues of sex and society, and mortality, the material they might not have otherwise had to deal with at this stage in their lives. For some it retriggered buried issues from their past. I realized by their horror that as much as this was about personal growth, we host disease on behalf of family systems as well as the over-culture. This notion created a level of detachment, albeit deflective, which was an important rational response to crisis. This psychic buffer gave me the space to begin to investigate my own core values, my thoughts, feelings, and behaviors, to see how those were reflected and/or denied in the society I lived in. This was just before the meds came. People still did not know much. There was hope on the horizon but we were left to make our own meanings because it seemed no one had meanings to offer. In retrospect, this was not true. Like many men I didn't have the resources or the support or the courage to access greater meaning. I was, however, able to ask questions. "How is living with HIV necessary for my growth as a gay man?" This was a dangerous question in light of the horrific losses happening in our community.

Being able to grasp the tension of paradox was important. Paradox, the dynamic tension between equal and opposite truths, can bring us to where the horrors and joys of life ultimately coexist. "What is the cost of this disease to me, my friends and family, society? What new skills must I learn? Where do I belong? How am I benefitting from this unwanted experience of the virus? How can confronting death heal me? How does my healing help others?" I later realized these were initiatory style questions.

Initiation radically separates us from former identities and goals; it separates us from preconceived notions of whom and what we once were and what the world once meant to us. I began to investigate how a rite of passage works.

The first stage of initiation, in this case, the diagnosis, catapults us into a lost kingdom. Often we are ripped away from much of what we know and love. We enter the realm of soul, a place few recognize because society denies the descent this represents. We enter a liminal space. We are neither here nor there. We are caught between our former and future selves. This effectively creates a psychic death, inevitably preparing us for our physical death.

The second stage is riddled with ordeals. It necessarily scars us. We are marked by the ordeal. Despite denial and avoidance we are taken deeper and forced to act. We are tested beyond our known capabilities. Again, society attempts to normalize crisis, but this only casts the initiate further out to the edge, into lonelier landscapes. We attempt to apply what we thought we knew, but this rarely works. Affliction requires us to develop new skills. As a caregiver I learned to become a fierce advocate in a sea of white coats. My own illness demanded new skills, seemingly counterproductive to mainstream ideas of progress. These skills included rest, learning to express deeper feelings, identifying real needs, taking the risk to ask for help. These new attitudes and skills can be severely tested upon our return to health.

The third stage, the return journey, is often overlooked because it can be the hardest to bear. Can we ever truly return to our former life when the process of healing has so drastically changed us? Can we uphold this new level of inner sovereignty and authority when others want us to be the same person they once knew? And yet for change to be fully integrated it requires a witnessing, an acknowledgment and appreciation for the journey taken, a mirroring back by the community to the initiate that she is now altered. The other parts of the system, some family and friends, have not undergone this journey. They may fail to recognize or appreciate the initiate's change, or may actively resist it out of their own fear or denial. Ideally, we respect and learn from the struggle and suffering of others. This is healthy evolution. This is what community needs the initiate to do, to return transformed, to show the rest, the uninitiated, the inner nature of change. For the rest, in turn, they too must mourn their losses before they can fully celebrate such hard-won success. The work of the initiate serves to bolster others' courage when the time for change calls upon them to face uncertainty.

GRS: Why is the concept of initiation important to our collective health?

RB: Initiation provides a cultural framing device for life-altering experiences. It inspires us to make meaning in the face of chaos. It revitalizes systems. Many people benefit when we create events where suffering is acknowledged and change is celebrated. When we deny soul we deny forces that revitalize. Where initiation patterns often fail is when we do not acknowledge, let alone celebrate, change. Denial perpetuates stress. A wise community recognizes the impact, and rewards of, change. Change is hard, not an enemy. When ignored that which wants to evolve but is denied reenters the separation/ordeal stages at more painful levels. This is true of the individual as it is in culture.

For example, HIV medications arrived in 1997. Suddenly those fortunate people, like my friends and I, started to *not* die of AIDS. There was so much to celebrate. It never happened. There were many complications in the medication process, but really the queer community was nearly decimated. It was too much for too many. Much of the heroism got lost in an unbearable ocean of grief. Survivors had to walk away. More than ever we needed society to be proud of such superhuman efforts. It never happened. So much lost.

For the sake of another future, let's imagine this occurred! The queer community and our extraordinary culture-changing allies were witnessed for their genius at the time of unfathomable loss. Everyone who needed medications got them. The world stood up with loving gratitude to acknowledge the amazing changes made to health care for the benefit of everyone. ACT UP's and the San Francisco model of health care internationally celebrated! Survivors, the nurses and doctors, the janitors, the grieving families, the army of friends and lovers, the remaining infected, witnessed and provided resources to heal. Younger gay men would have seen how much healthy pride we have in ourselves and in one another. Battle scars touched, and one day, if not soothed, stilled. Such massive healing occurred. Young gay men would have wanted to be part of the movement rather than push it away in fear and self-disgust as it happens today. Our communities would still be a community as a result of healing. Imagine the exceptional wisdom, such truly great collective knowledge that could then have been mobilized for the rest of the world. And in this fantasy this virus would not be the global pandemic it is today where so many power brokers continue to greedily put their heads in the tar sands. And the trauma gets buried deeper, costs humanity more, sets the stakes up higher for generations to come to bear. No leader ever apologized for doing nothing for five years.

We need to know what is worth healing for. Acknowledged survivors, those marked by extraordinary change, thrive. Initiation promotes personal and cultural value.

Globally, we need adaptability and resilience. We must anchor ourselves in the spirit of change. We are in a massive global initiation process. Countercultural movements recognize the miasma of our shared crisis. As a mythic and imaginative construct, initiation tells us where to look next. When in crisis get help. Offer help. Adapt. Share. History does show examples that people can be at their best in crisis. We need to acknowledge that we are in crisis first. The fact that we don't shows us the level of desensitization we have endured. This includes for most denial of our unearned privilege, of class, race, gender, or other ranks we hold.

Using the construct of illness as a rite of passage would lead us to ask relevant questions: How is my cancer diagnosis related to this world that cries out for change? How does it relate to a collective experience? For my uncle it was, "Wow, ten people on my block have cancer; I remember fifteen years ago when they used that empty lot at the end of our block as a toxic waste site." When we make connections with our private experiences to the larger picture, our healthy anger can lead us to taking collective action.

When we claim our personal and collective agency new roles emerge. We might become wounded healers or healer-activists. Psychologically, when we can ask hard but loving questions like, "How might my world need me to heal now?" we begin to move out of personalizing blame and shame and see the necessity of illness as an initiatory function that has the potential to benefit others now and in the future.

GRS: I grow so tired of the idea that we get sick because we've done something wrong, that we are bad people.

RB: Exactly, that is a meme rooted in fear, entrenched by religion, and profited by the industrial medical model. Illness is suffering that connects us to the world, one that might give us a glimpse of beauty that we may have never known. It asks us to care, to evolve, to reimagine health from the perspective of interconnected wellness. Illness evolves humanity.

GRS: What are the side effects of a world where people don't value initiation? What do you see as the major barriers to including these practices in the world we live in?

RB: From a neutral perspective, it doesn't matter. Magic is afoot. We are in a time of unprecedented exposure. What is repressed leaks sideways. What was hidden is revealed. Greater crises are erupting all around us. There are no guarantees, only more uncertainty. This is the stuff of initiation. From the ozone layer to the Internet, boundaries are dissolving because we have a much wider, albeit dizzying, understanding of the nature of life, if not death.

GRS: What do you think would change in the world if the concept of initiation became integrated in our culture or available within our systems of medicine? For instance, what would be altered if people could choose to code the survival of cancer as a kind of initiation process as an important factor in their recommendations for the treatment of illness?

RB: Anyone who survives cancer knows they are a different person on the other side of it—different although they may not be able to fully articulate how or why. A famous homeopath and physician by the name of Whitmont said growth happens between the dramatic interplay of willingness and resistance. Paradox, again. Yes, we want to get better, but we naturally and necessarily resist change. Again, change is a primary role and function illness plays; it pushes us to places we would rather not go. Illness is inherently not bad; it can be our ally. As in the concept of the shamanic, the otherworldly, the underworld place illness takes us, illness can be an ally we must wrestle with, to the near death, in order to gain its awesome powers.

This awesome struggle leads to a psychic death of that which no longer serves us. In the space left behind we gain a renewed understanding of ourselves in our world. We feel empowered to act, to participate in the changes that are happening within and around us. We experience a vitality we may never have known before. We can bring this understanding to a much larger scale and truly know that we are part of something bigger than our former limited concept of self and spirit.

In the mundane sense, illness forces us to ritualize our life with pills and appointments. Illness, however, can also be an ecstatic container, a crucible within which to let go and temporarily forget who we once were. Think of the ill person temporarily turned rabid or wild. This is a frightening form of the ecstatic. To see it as a rite of passage, illness can become a catalyst within which our lives can be forever altered, sometimes for the best. Many people describe to me and other healers that their journey through illnesses is the greatest gift they have ever experienced.

GRS: It may only take the healer introducing or suggesting it...

RB: As healthcare providers, healers, and caregivers we can gently suggest or even look for the holistic understanding of initiatory patterns. For instance, when a patient is raging, rather than taking it personally, we can recognize a death cycle has begun, and listen closer for clues of the healing grief that wants out. We can also invite people to celebrate their hard-won successes, and introduce nondenominational, ritual-like processes that witness the path undertaken. Seen from a systems perspective, we can reflect on our own past *interrupted* initiations and continue to do our inner and outer work. This helps us have empathy and compassion and importantly to not unconsciously resent or rely on the sick person to be our scapegoat, to do our psychological work for us. Ultimately we are learning to give ourselves and each other healthy attention. This is how we know who we are and who we can become.

GRS: What is your offering to these interesting times in terms of your work? What does the world/what do humans need most right now in order to return to a healthy culture?

RB: As a facilitator, counselor, artist, and teacher I cocreate temporary spaces where positive risk and vulnerability can occur, opportunities to share caring containers of health-promoting attention, from a mother's hug to large community healing rituals, to helping people imagine policies and laws that protect people and the natural world from social injustice. I work with issues around gender and sexuality. I help people find resiliency from trauma. I also create events that help us rethink how we can play our way into community. We need our own tribe, people with whom we can share our stories. We need spaces to gather and reconsider what kind of culture we want. Otherwise there is little consciousness in change, only reaction, potentially violent reaction at that, where risk and vulnerability are experienced in isolation, as negative rather than life-inspiring forces.

As my mentor Ed Wolf, longtime AIDS educator, gifted story-teller, and magical activist, says, "Amnesty. We need to give ourselves and each other a break. We need places where we can ventilate and be validated." This is so miraculously simple, so profoundly loving. If we temporarily relax concepts of right and wrong, we glimpse from the corner of our heart that just maybe everything is playing its part for evolution to occur. With more awareness comes new ideas and together we evolve. Initiation requires and induces conscious awareness.

I offer personal support and group retreats to explore illness as a rite of passage. The journey taken together becomes a refuge from well-meaning others who have not yet stepped through this gateway of susceptibility. And yet, births and deaths are givens. We all need a team to be on. Finding the right team or tribe is one of life's other great challenges. Illness helped me find mine.

GRS: Can you say more about the role of celebration, responsibility, and service that are the next phases in the initiatory process?

RB: Celebration is necessary. It's the birthday party with soul; a rebirthing, a giving birth to ourselves through the pain of crisis and letting ourselves be witnessed. As a Western cultural reframe, we must move through many layers of debilitating guilt and self-pity into the experience of self-empathy. We become resensitized to our lived experiences. With self-empathy, we authentically extend empathy to the world. This is an example of how wounded healers, which many of us are, can reframe crisis as necessary and ultimately health stimulating. "Go ahead and bitch until you cry. You are worthy. We see your pain and desire. You are wanted and needed by this crazy world in the ways you wish to offer your gifts." Our pain matures into wisdom, which seasons us to be fully present for others' growth, too.

After an initiation we take on new roles and responsibilities. Cancer survivors raise money, become volunteers, go and speak to current patients, become advocates. I am now the gay men's health coordinator for Vancouver Island, BC, something I never imagined doing. When I cocreated an event on December 1, 2011, World AIDS Day, to mark thirty years of AIDS, it was a soulful, celebratory event of the kind that most of us never participated in. In a gentle ritual format thirty people from many walks of life took the stage and spoke, sang, or danced their story. It felt like we and the others lost to this disease were brought back into community.

At the end of my partner's two-year struggle with cancer we got married. Gay marriage in Canada had been only recently legalized. Politically, I was opposed to the historical meaning of marriage, but my anger that other queer folk were not being allowed to demonstrate their love compelled me to propose. He said yes. We had survived. In my spontaneous vows I said, "I thought I was going to lose you." We turned to see a couple hundred people openly weeping. We celebrated his, our common, return to life; we were magically touched by the symbolic, a triumphant wedding at the end of an era-changing battle. And what a beautiful ritual it was. It was bigger than us. It was about our small rural community fighting for his life. It was about our nation's laws evolving. The spirit of celebration claimed us for its own. Years later, one young gay neighbor daringly said, "But, of course, he's the happy AIDS patient." My husband now helps so many others more courageously enter their own dark night.

On a sadder note, we exist in the most death phobic society that humanity has ever seen. I saw a picture set in LA where there was a drive-by funeral. People didn't even get out of their cars! The concept of death as celebration is a healthy part of the mourning process. Death is not a failure, it is a given. Illness as initiation brings us to health or death but neither is a failure. Both can refresh systems. It can be about grieving and finding the joy in what we truly value.

Applying the idea of initiation to health care gives us more power as healers and people going through healing to take necessary risks. Using this construct of initiation refreshes the social system. This is the equal and opposite function. Celebration is the twin to the crisis of illness. Both are sacred. Both bring the personal and collective to a greater state of awareness. Because there is no money in celebrating healing or initiation, North American society is locked in a financial leg-hold where illness pays more than health does. We must return to the sacred as a way to connect to the Body Erotic. The system crumbles on its way to wholeness. Chaos before change, said Jung. The English word *holy* comes to us all the way from the eleventh-century Old English word *hālig*, derived from *hāl*, meaning whole. In my heart and body, in my most rational senses, I know we are one another's holy.

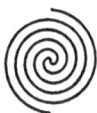

Conclusion

With our lives we will make our answers all the time,
to this ravenous, beautiful, mutilated, gorgeous world.

— Victoria Safford

Today the sun shines, the rhododendrons are laughing, and everything is in bloom. I feel blessed and bless everything I see. This is the way I wish it always was between people and places. It is easy to believe we are meant to be here and healing our lives is possible. We can have a different kind of existence, another chance at health.

Sometimes modern life sucks us dry, like a spigot placed over our hearts to drain life force from us. It's up to us to refill our body, mind, and spirit with service and joy. The truth is that every human wants to belong, to celebrate, to love, and to be safe.

Humans do terrible things when we feel threatened. Many people have a low tolerance for uncertain times. The fear of the unknown acts as a bonding agent. But when we bond through fear or complaint about what we feel is the cause of our problems, we can find a scapegoat or join in mob mentality. This prevents us from empathy, connection and the possibility of finding a new perspective.

Healers of the present day will find ourselves in situations where people are becoming rigid in their fears about what is coming next. We can use all these sacred healing practices to remind people we are living with or serving that they are not alone. There are always possibilities to relax, connect, and transform suffering. Just ask a wounded healer.

There are so many other methods we can employ in order to meet each other and solve the problems that we face. It takes time to build true intimacy and relationship, but it is work worth doing. The world seems to be starving for magic and wonder, for hope and healing. It is crucial to join others to bring spirit back into our lives.

Joanna Macy and Chris Johnstone outline some strategies for facing fear in their book *Active Hope: How to Face the Mess We're In Without Going Crazy.* They challenge people to find more reasonable measures of success, defining success as "that which contributes to the well-being of our world" and invite us to celebrate the victory of each step toward this goal. [1]

When we have hope, we risk disappointment. When we inspire hope, we risk that others may be disappointed. Macy and Johnstone offer an alternative called "active hope." This is the kind of hope that is a personal practice. It involves creating a best-case scenario for the future, breaking it down into manageable actions and dedicating ourselves to the small steps which will bring it into being. [2]

The idea that we can always see our effectiveness is not realistic and perhaps part of the instant gratification culture that we are attempting to revise. If we are lucky, our patient recovers, the kids we teach learn something, and our counseling client feels better. In the best case scenario, we make a visible difference we can acknowledge. Those are great moments, but our attachment to having them happen frequently is not always advantageous. Sometimes we have to do the work that is directly in front of us and never get to see the results of our actions. Instead, the challenge is to trust that our children, students, or some descendent in the future may be touched by what we do. [3] We can continue to support each other and hold the vision we pray for; there is no certainty about where we are going. Perhaps all we can do is exactly what is in front of us and contribute as much as possible to the joy of the new world unfolding around us. Both receiving and providing healing have so often been viewed as intensely personal, even isolating experiences. It may be that this kind of loneliness is drastically outdated.

The journey back to health must be walked together.

It is time to question what we want to be central and vital to our health as a culture and begin to live the true answers to those questions. If global revolutionary healers lead the way, a true revolution of the spirit can begin. We will stop committing collective suicide and begin to live as if our bodies mattered, grounded in the cycles of a place, in the health of our soil. We will treat each other with respect. We will make our daily and seasonal rituals meaningful and inspirational and connect with the larger source of everything. We will call our fragmented selves back home and create personal practices that return us to our values and priorities. We will honor the voices of our shadows so that we don't act unconsciously from our hurt egos. We will remember to listen to our dreams. We will allow alchemical miracles to happen as our wounds become our greatest gifts. We will travel the path of initiation when it finds us and take our teachings into the world to serve our communities. Even as imperfect, wounded healers, we affect positive cultural transformation.

I want to be fierce about the emerging world and I want you to imagine it with me. How can it be beautiful instead of horrible? How will we bring the parts of ourselves and our culture back together? How do we stop inappropriately nursing fear and open ourselves to new possibilities? How do we stand up to institutions that keep us mired in dis-ease and separate from the planet? How can we dream larger, for more than just ourselves and our families? What does it mean to reengage in a web of life that includes all beings in our definition of collective health care?

As healers and changers of culture, we are strong advocates for the people we support who are already eager to do this work. We don't have to convert anyone to a religion or pretend to be authorities in traditions in which we have not earned expertise. We journey with our patients, clients, colleagues, communities and students. We reflect their courage, and create space for Spirit to come into our meetings or sessions. We can also allow ourselves to integrate our understanding of the spiritual practices of the world into our healing work. Let's firmly move past any residual fear of being labeled as a witch or charlatan. People are hungry and we have knowledge to share and a clear invitation to share it. It is time to take a holy risk and invite the sacred back into our personal work and our healing practices.

I dare you to commune with folks with whom you may not have obvious things in common and express solidarity by offering your skills to their needs. This might take a while. Please stay with it and build relationships with people that you don't interact with in daily life. Respect is a shared language.

Daring to stay alive means there can still be surprises. Every breath is a new world, the initiation of a desire for healing. The deepest inspiration comes in the dark space between events or around the fire when we sing or drum or create. The truth touches us when there are no more distractions. We reach across the isolation of our culture to hold each other and remember what has been lost or found. The new forms will come but now we become quiet enough to touch the dark stream and make more sacred space.

Divesting of hope is ludicrous. Our excessive Western lifestyles are not sustainable in the face of a planet warming, melting, transforming into something that we have never seen before. In every country, people aspire to Western culture's levels of spending, technology, disposable income, stress, leisure and we equate that privilege with freedom. We know that ever increasing consumption is not freedom, but it is difficult to stop. We know in our bones that we have the power to change this outcome. We are hard wired to give, to connect, to live better with less. We will make our way back to connected tribes and practical relationship with land. We will help each other remember our non-human family because of who we are on the inside. All the false social training that we receive cracks, chips and flakes eventually. In the emergencies, we rise. We tend to harmony. We seek each other. We will make this turning one way or another.

What is the role of the global healer in these times? We surely invigorate the places where we know that we belong, where we suspect that we can create joy. We bring life to old wounds when we dare to love beyond measure, when we gather our power and revision the world to come. I would rather be cracked open than sealed shut. I want our desires and concerns to enkindle our greatest pride so that we can find the healing ways by which we will live. We are in a battle for our collective imagination and health, a war about who gets to decide what's real. Our healing is stronger than the media's messages that fear is all we need. It's time to dream the beginning of the world instead of the end.

I dare you.

Here we go.

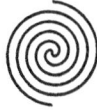

Contributors

Robert Birch, MA, is an interdisciplinary wellness practitioner. His work generates cultural processes and products such as nature-based retreats, performance art, photojournalism, activism, and educational events. He considers himself blessed to have had a number of key mentors and friends in his life who have helped him grow, watched him fall, and inspired him to heal. He began his first theatre company at age fifteen. He taught drama in education workshops in colleges at the age of seventeen. Over the past thirty years Robert has been recognized as a caregiver, farmer, lived on welfare, and struggled with his addictive personality.

He has served as a social justice and community health educator and curriculum writer. He likes to rant as an activist, journalist, and performance artist. He often says he wears invisible platform pumps that double as his soapbox. He loves his work as a peer counselor, conference organizer and trainer for regional, national, and international projects. He is a leading applied theatre practitioner of Playback Theatre with a rich history of public performance, community arts-based research, and social development. Last year he was awarded the Queer Educator of the Year by the Victoria, BC, gay community. He is also one of five active international facilitators of a weeklong training for men who love men, developed by Harry Hay, the historic founder of the modern LGBT movement. While continuing to write queer HIV/AIDS narratives, his future goals include initiating a much overdue local AIDS memorial, advocating for a provincial gay men's health strategy, and codesigning a queer mobile health and community performance art clinic to helps us reenvision health as an experience of community, with a lot of help from his friends.

He is a regular contributor to the online magazine Positive Lite (positivelite.com). Visit robertbirch.ca.

Jalaja (pronounced DJA-la-dja) **Bonheim, Ph.D**., is an internationally acclaimed speaker, teacher, and author. Raised in Austria and Germany, she spent several years in India, immersed in the study of Indian temple dance, mythology, and spirituality.

Today she is one of the foremost experts in the use of circle gatherings as a tool for empowering women and healing individuals and communities. She is the founder and director of the Institute for Circlework (instituteforcirclework.org) and has trained hundreds of Circlework leaders in America, Canada, and the Middle East, including ministers, teachers, social workers, psychotherapists, and corporate executives.

Jalaja Bonheim is the author of five books, including *The Hunger for Ecstasy: Fulfilling the Soul's Need for Intimacy and Passion* and *Aphrodite's Daughters: Women's Sexual Stories and the Journey of the Soul*. Based on the stories of ordinary American women, *Aphrodite's Daughters* explores the central role of sexuality in women's spiritual journey and has changed the lives of thousands of women.

Growing up as a Jew in postwar Germany, Bonheim's lifelong inquiry into the causes of human violence and the journey of healing and transformation come from this devastating legacy of war. Since 2005, she has traveled regularly to Israel and Palestine, where she empowers Jewish and Palestinian women to serve as agents of peace and healing in their communities.

In her latest book, *Evolving Toward Peace: Awakening the Global Heart,* which is garnering rave reviews, she shares her insights into the nature of the collective journey of transformation we are currently engaged in. With dozens of stories from her work with peacemakers around the world, she shows how today millions are awakening to a new consciousness.

Visit jalajabonheim.com and instituteforcirclework.org.

Jamie Seraphina Capranos is a full-time clinican in a busy office primarily prescribing classical homeopathy and Western herbs. She is a third-generation herbalist and energyworker, and feels blessed to have had her mother and grandparents as her first teachers. It took eight years of practicing until she finally gave herself full permission to come "out" to her patients as an energy healer. Now she whole-heartedly attends to her patients' chronic and acute illnesses as much as to their spiritual crises and fractured energetic membranes.

At the age of sixteen she suffered a serious injury to her spine that led the medical profession to conclude she would live a life in chronic pain. Determined to heal herself, she returned to her roots and began a professional study of natural medicine. While she has spent her career studying in formal colleges, she has equally found herself in unexpected apprenticeships with indigenous medicine women and wise healers. She feels deeply nourished by both the scientific and spiritual sides of medicine, and in fact finds them dif-ferent languages expressing the very same conclusion—that life is the expression of the divinely arranged intelligence of nature. Alongside a busy practice, she teaches herbalism and homeopathy internation-ally. Her classes are known for being empowering, earth-based, and rooted in spirit. She has been published extensively in health maga-zines and journals, and is a regular guest teacher at universities and colleges in British Columbia. Visit jamiecapranos.com.

Lorie Eve Dechar is an alchemist, acupuncturist, artist, psycho-therapist, and explorer of consciousness. Her first commitment is to healing—personal, interpersonal and planetary. After that, there is bridging the space between the divine and daily worlds. Next comes beauty, paradox, and poetry. And then there is love.

Lorie is the author of *Five Spirits: Alchemical Acupuncture for Psychological and Spiritual Healing*. With her husband and life inspirer Benjamin Fox, she envisioned and cocreated the Alchem-ical Healing Mentorship, a training program for acupuncturists, holistic healers, and other agents of change. She is on the faculty of Tri-State College of Acupuncture in NYC and is adjunct faculty at The Acupuncture Academy in Leamington Spa, UK. In addition, she teaches regularly at the Esalen Institute in Big Sur, California, and shows up to practice alchemy wherever there's a chunk of lead, a suitable laboratory, and apprentices who want to learn.

For the past twenty-five years, Lorie has danced around the ques-tion of how human beings heal and transform. Through her work with individuals and with groups, she seeks to find ways to inspire people to become more of who they truly are, to recognize their own divinity, and to honor the darkness as well as the light in the healing process.

When she isn't off traveling, Lorie lives by the sea in Downeast Maine with Benjamin and Professor, the black and white cat. She tends to the spirits in the garden, woods, and islands and is currently stirring the cauldron of a second book on alchemy. Visit fivespirits.com.

Isa Gucciardi, Ph.D., holds degrees and certificates in transpersonal psychology, cultural and linguistic anthropology, comparative religion, hypnotherapy, and transformational healing. She has spent over thirty years studying spiritual, therapeutic, and meditative techniques from around the world. She has worked with master teachers of Buddhism, Christianity, Judaism, and Sufism, as well as expert shamanic practitioners from the traditions of Hawaii, indigenous North and South America, Siberia, and Nepal.

Isa is the creator of Depth Hypnosis, a groundbreaking therapeutic model that has won rave reviews from psychotherapeutic and spiritual counselors alike. She has published numerous articles, been featured in several documentaries, and she is widely quoted by healing professionals working in a diverse array of healing modalities. She is also the Founding Director of the Foundation of the Sacred Stream, a nonprofit organization and resource center where she offers trainings in Depth Hypnosis, Applied Shamanism, Buddhist Psychology Studies, Integrated Energy Medicine, Destination Studies, and Transpersonal Studies.

Dr. Gucciardi speaks five languages, and has lived in eleven countries. In addition to directing and teaching at the Foundation of the Sacred Stream and the Sacred Stream Center in Berkeley, CA, she maintains an active Depth Hypnosis and Applied Shamanism healing practice in San Francisco. Well loved by her students for her insight, humor, and passion for teaching, Dr. Isa Gucciardi serves groups of students throughout the United States and abroad. Visit sacredstream.org.

Anne Hill, D.Min., writes, teaches, and speaks widely on dreams, spirituality, and publishing. She is coauthor with Starhawk and Diane Baker of *Circle Round: Raising Children in Goddess Traditions*, and was active in Reclaiming, a feminist spirituality community, beginning in the mid-1980s. In 2012 she published an ebook about her experiences, *The Baby and the Bathwater: What I learned About Spirituality, Magic, Community, Ecstasy, and Power from 25 Years in Reclaiming.*

Anne's essays, music, and poetry have been published in several anthologies and periodicals, including *The Pagan Book of Living and Dying* and the *Encyclopedia of Religion and Nature*, *Mothering* magazine, and the *New Age Journal*. She was profiled in the book *Modern Pagans*, and is currently a columnist for *SageWoman Magazine*.

In 1992 Anne started Serpentine Music, serpentinemusic. com, to introduce and distribute music to the growing nature religions movement. She produced six albums including *Circle Round and Sing!* and *The Best of Pagan Song*, and distributed hundreds of titles worldwide until 2010. Today Serpentine Music & Media is Anne's publishing hub, distributing her several self-published titles including *What To Do When Dreams Go Bad: A Practical Guide to Nightmares*.

Anne earned a Doctor of Ministry degree in 2003 at Wisdom University, and was the first graduate of Dr. Jeremy Taylor's Marin Institute for Projective Dreamwork in 2002. She is on the faculty of Cherry Hill Seminary, where she teaches Dreams in Spiritual Direction to M.Div. students. She earned a black belt in aikido in 2003.

In 1994 Anne began advising authors on Internet marketing, and in 2005 she started her award-winning Blog o' Gnosis, gnosiscafe.com/gcblog. Anne also writes for her consulting practice Creative Content Coaching, creativecontentcoaching.com, as well as the Huffington Post and O'Reilly Media's Tools of Change for Publishing blog.

In 2008 Anne founded Dream Talk Radio, dreamtalkradio.net, a weekly radio show, podcast, and now a YouTube channel, youtube. com/user/dreamtalkradio, where she interviews leading thinkers about dreams, transformation, and society. Anne also interviews leaders in publishing, and is a specialist in author platforms. She currently educates authors in building their web presence, and is at work on several books.

Anne has three grown children, and resides in Bodega Bay, CA.

Dawn Isidora works with individuals, couples, and groups as a spiritual mentor and educator, exploring lives and relationships through a holistic, spiritual lens. Much of Dawn's work is informed by the wisdom of the five Sacred Elements: Air (thought, communication, and respiration), Fire (will, creativity, and digestion), Water (emotion, dreams, and circulation), Earth (home, livelihood, and musculoskeletal), and Spirit (connection, integration, and nervous system) as portals of discovery to each soul's unique blueprint. She also looks to these Elements as diagnostic tools to reveal hidden strengths and imbalances.

Depending upon each individualized situation, there are many tools from which Dawn draws: discussion, emotional exploration, guided meditation and trance (also called hypnosis), neurolin-guistic programming (NLP, used to shift thought and behavior patterns), yogic sets, or meditations. She assists clients to discover their own spiritual paths, build a personalized practice that works for their lives, strengthen their relationships with mystery, improve relationships with other humans, integrate life's transitions big and small, clarify communications, and embrace the sexual self as part of a healthy spiritual whole. She welcomes people of all genders, orientations, backgrounds, and histories, as well as diversity of race, religion, and economic circumstance.

Dawn's intent is to support her clients and students in forging grounded, authentic relationships with themselves, their beloveds, their communities, and the Mysterious Ones. She holds certifi-cation in conflict mediation, hypnotherapy, and Kundalini Yoga instruction. As an internationally recognized teacher and workshop facilitator, she has worked in the spiritual and self-empowerment movement for twenty-five years and through the magic of Skype, has clients spread across the globe.

Dawn teaches regularly in the Pacific Northwest, as well as at a variety of retreats and intensives around the world. Visit dawn-isidora.com.

Starhawk is the author or coauthor of twelve books, including *The Spiral Dance: A Rebirth of the Ancient Religion of the Great Goddess*, the now-classic ecotopian novel, *The Fifth Sacred Thing, The Earth Path: Grounding Your Spirit in the Rhythms of Nature,* and her latest, *The Empowerment Manual: A Guide for Collaborative Groups*, about power and process for horizontal, directly democratic organizing.

Starhawk is a founder, director, and core teacher for Earth Activist Trainings, which are intensive seminars that combine per-maculture design, effective activism, and earth-based spirituality. With ten years of experience in permaculture design and teach-ing, she has pioneered the application of permaculture principles to social organizations, policy, and strategy. Since its first course in May of 2001, Earth Activist Trainings have graduated over five hundred students who now shepherd projects that range from community power-down strategies in Iowa City to water catchment programs in Bolivia, from inner-city gardens in San Francisco to women's programs in the West Bank of Palestine. Starhawk's own expertise is in the communication of permaculture's systems thinking through images, writing, and innovative teaching techniques. She also maintains active permaculture models in both her San Francisco city garden and her west Sonoma County ranch. Visit earthactivisttraining.org.

In 1973, she won the Samuel Goldwyn Creative Writing Award at UCLA, where she was a graduate student in film. She cowrote the first two documentaries, *Goddess Remembered* and *Burning Times*, in the Women and Spirituality trilogy produced by the National Film Board of Canada and directed by Donna Read in the late eighties, and wrote the commentary for the third, *Full Circle*. The trilogy remained in the top ten of sales and rentals for the Film Board for over a decade.

She and Donna Read formed Belili Productions in 1992 to make documentaries on women and the earth. They produced *Signs Out of Time*, a documentary on the life and work of archaeologist Marija Gimbutas, in 2004, and released *Permaculture: The Growing Edge* in 2010. Visit www.belili.org.

A committed activist for peace, global justice, and the environment, and most recently for the Occupy Wall Street movement, she travels globally teaching, lecturing, and training in permaculture, spirituality, organizing, group dynamics, and facilitation. Starhawk's archives are maintained by the Graduate Theological Union Library in Berkeley, California. Visit starhawk.org.

Suzanne Sterling is a dedicated musician, yogi, activist, and social innovator who has been performing and teaching transformational workshops for over twenty-five years. She is an ecstatic vocalist, innovative teacher, and invoker of the sacred. A leading expert in sound and consciousness, Suzanne brings a unique perspective to her work in the world. Taking all on a passionate, ecstatic journey into the heart of creativity, authentic connection with Source, and joyful service.

Suzanne has been a featured artist/teacher at numerous national and international festivals and conferences such as Wanderlust (North America), Omega Institute, Esalen, Kripalu, Yoga

Journal, Hanuman, Tadasana, Burning Man, Ecstatic Dance, Bhaktifest, Boomfest, Lightning in a Bottle, and Earthdance, where she led the world's largest Spiral Dance for five thousand people.

Suzanne is a certified yoga instructor whose unique style enriches numerous nationally recognized teacher training programs and certifications. She is an integral part of the nationwide faculty for Yogaworks, Moksha Yoga-Chicago, and Laughing Lotus-NYC.

Since 2007 she has been training leaders of conscious activism through her cofounded (with Seane Corn and Hala Khouri) organization Off The Mat, Into the World (OTM). OTM uses the power of yoga to ignite grassroots social change. Currently Suzanne is the Director of OTM's Seva Challenge, which has raised over three million dollars for organizations in Cambodia, Africa, Haiti, and India.

As a ritual designer and priestess, she has worked with acclaimed author and activist Starhawk and the international Reclaiming Community, creating ritual and training teachers in eco-feminist spirituality. These trainings and intensives have been taught nationally in California, Oregon, and Vermont.

An award-winning musician, she has released five solo albums and five DVD soundtracks. All of her music is available from her website and on iTunes.

Suzanne's life work is dedicated to inspiring others to find their unique voice and to use self-expression as a tool for community building and conscious evolution. She is the founder of Voice of Change.

Find out more at suzannesterling.com or on Facebook and Twitter.

To learn more about the mission and vision of Off the Mat, Into the World, visit offthematintotheworld.org.

END NOTES

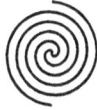

Introduction

1. Julia Cameron, *The Artist's Way* (New York, NY:Tarcher/Putnam, 1992), 1.
2. Claire Hoertz Bardaracco, *Prescribing Faith* (Waco, TX: Baylor University, 2007), 92: It is important to notice how many risks scientists have taken to "prove" that health is influenced by factors other than the pure cause and effect of a single variable on another.
3. Ibid.
4. Ibid.
5. Gregory P. Fields, *Religious Therapeutics: Body and Health in Yoga, Ayurveda, and Tantra* (Albany, NY: State University of New York, 2001), 3.

A Tale of a Spiritual Seeker

1. It is both my belief and my sincere hope that our society has evolved to include a worldview where religious education can move beyond literalism, expanding our ability to hold all teachings as both a kind of truth and wider storied wisdom. When we can look at all religion with both a critical and creative mind, perhaps we will get somewhere.
2. A Google search on 2/4/13 for "reasons not to kill yourself" yielded 9,380,000 results on the Internet including a brilliant blog on Huffington Post by Eliot Schrefer that lists "Your teeth are made in stars" and "Many, many creatures are depending on you" in his article: "5 Scientific Reasons not to Kill Yourself." www.huffingtonpost.com/eliot-schrefer/five-scientific-reasons-n_b_126526.html.

3. Forward thinking psychiatrists are now combining many adjunct treatments to the medication they prescribe for patients, incorporating art and music lessons, occupational therapies, acupuncture, meditation, movement, gym memberships, body-based psychotherapies, and other myriad paths to holistic health.
4. K. Chimm Wong, *History of Chinese Medicine* (New York, NY: AMS Press, 1973), 46.
5. Five Elements Chart. chineseacupuncturehealing.com/wp-content/uploads/2011/03/THE-5-elements.png.
6. K. Chimm Wong, *History of Chinese Medicine* (New York, NY: AMS Press, 1973), xxv.
7. Fruehauf Heiner, Science, Politics and the Making of TCM: chineseclassics.org/j/images/tcmcrisis.pdf.
8. Articles published in 1958 from Heiner source.
9. See a series of articles published in 1958 in China's official newspaper, Renmin Ribao (The Peoples' Daily); i.e., "Dali kaizhan xiyi xuexi zhongyi yundong" (Let Us Give Strong Momentum to the Western Doctors Studying Chinese Medicine Movement). See Yu Zhenchu, Zhongguo Yixue Jianshi (A Brief History of Chinese Medical Science), Fuzhou: Fujian Kexue Jishu, 1983, p. 446.
10. K. Chimm Wong, *History of Chinese Medicine* (New York, NY: AMS Press, 1973), 41.
11. International Institute of Chinese Medicine, professional medical oath taken at graduation, August 2002.

Body and Mind, Soul and Spirit

1. James Hillman, *A Blue Fire* (New York: Harper and Row, 1991), 118.
2. James Hillman, *A Psyche The Size of the Earth*, essay in *Ecopsychology* (New York: Sierra Club Books, 1995), xvii.
3. quoting Koenig, Claire Hoertz Bardaracco, *Prescribing Faith* (Waco, TX: Baylor University, 2007), 143.
4. As of 2011, the Midwives Alliance of North America (MANA), mana.org/statechart.html, identifies Alabama, District of Columbia, Illinois, Indiana, Iowa, Kentucky, Maryland, North Carolina, Pennsylvania, and South Carolina as states where midwifery is illegal; Georgia and Hawaii as states where the practice of midwifery is legal but there is no licensure; and Connecticut,

Nebraska, Ohio, and West Virginia as states where there is no law forbidding midwifery but no legal protection for midwives.

5. Anne Llewellyn Barstow, *Witchcraze: A New History of the European Witch Hunts,* (San Francisco: Pandora HarperCollins, 1994), 160–164.
6. Gregory P. Fields, *Religious Therapeutics: Body and Health in Yoga, Ayurveda, and Tantra* (Albany, NY: State University of New York, 2001), 1.
7. Claire Hoertz Bardaracco, *Prescribing Faith* (Waco, TX: Baylor University, 2007), 144.
8. Ibid, p. 145.
9. Margaret Wills, *Connection, Action and Hope: An Invitation to Reclaim the "Spiritual" in Health Care* (Springer. Journal of Religion and Health, 2007), 424.
10. Sharts-Hopko 359 or Wills 426.
11. WHCCAMP 2 or Wills 426.
12. Margaret Wills, *Connection, Action, and Hope: An Invitation to Reclaim the "Spiritual" in Health Care* (Springer: Journal of Religion and Health, 2007), 428.
13. Ibid.
14. Kaiser 2000, p. 13 or Wills 429.
15. Kaiser 2000, p. 13 or Wills 429.

Embodiment

1. Wendy Palmer, *The Intuitive Body: Discovering the Wisdom of Conscious Embodiment and Aikido* (Berkeley, CA: Blue Snake Books, 1994), 23–26.
2. Eugene T. Gendlin, *Focusing* (New York, NY: Bantam Dell, 1981), 32–50.

Connection to Land

1. Joanna Macy and Molly Young Brown, *Coming Back to Life: Practices to Reconnect Our Lives, Our World* (Canada: New Society Publishing, 1998), 27–34.
2. Article on Civil Rights for Mother Earth, guardian.co.uk/environment/2011/apr/10/bolivia-enshrines-natural-worlds-rights.
3. David Abram, *Spell of the Sensuous: Perception and Language in a More-Than-Human World* (New York, NY: Pantheon Press, 1996), 145–149.

4. Stephen Harrod Buhner, *The Lost Language of Plants: The Ecological Importance of Plant Medicines for Life on Earth* (White River Junction, VT: Chelsea Green Publishing, 2002), 65.
5. Starhawk, *The Earth Path* (New York, NY: Harper Collins, 2004), 56–58.

Ritual

1. Margo Anand, *The Art of Everyday Ecstasy* (New York, NY: Broadway Books, 1998), 113–115.

Creativity and Ecstasy

1. Julia Cameron, *The Artist's Way* (New York, NY:Tarcher/Putnam, 1992), 3.
2. Jalaja Bonheim, *Hunger for Ecstasy* (Daybreak Press, 2001), 100–103.
3. Barbara Ehrenreich, *Dancing in the Streets* (London, England: Granta Publications, 2007), 179.
4. Ibid, pp. 172–179.
5. Joanna Macy, *Coming Back to Life: Practices to Reconnect Our Lives, Our World* (Canada: New Society Publishing, 1998), 59–60.

Soul Retrieval

1. Lorie Dechar, Alchemical Healing Mentorship, May 20–23, 2010, Portland, Oregon.
2. Caitlin and John Matthews, *Encyclopedia of Celtic Wisdom* (Shaftesbury, Dorset UK: Element Books, 1994), 299.
3. Ibid, pp. 299–303.
4. Peter Levine, *In an Unspoken Voice: How the Body Releases Trauma and Restores Goodness* (Berkeley, CA: North Atlantic Books), 137.
5. Ibid, p. 48.

Personal Practice

1. Joanna Macy and Chris Johnstone, *Active Hope* (Novato, CA: New World Library, 2012), 203–204.

Shadow and Dreams

1. David Richo, *Shadow Dance: Liberating the Power and Creativity of Your Dark Side* (Boston, MA: Shambala Publishing, 1999), 32.
2. Ibid, pp. 13.
3. Ibid, p. 25.
4. Jeremy Taylor, *The Living Labyrinth* (Mahway, NY: Paulist Press, 1998), 262–268.

Alchemy

1. Lorie Eve Dechar *Five Spirits* (2005), 138–142.
2. Ibid, p. 76.
3. James Hillman, *A Blue Fire* (New York: Harper and Row, 1991), 125-126.
4. December 16, 2011 11:49am by Barbara Ehrenreich and John Ehrenreich. *The Nation*.

Initiation

1. David Richo, *Shadow Dance: Liberating the Power and Creativity of Your Dark Side* (Boston, MA: Shambala Publishing, 1999), 64–65.

Conclusion

1. Joanna Macy and Chris Johnstone, *Active Hope* (Novato, CA: New World Library, 2012), 224.
2. Ibid, pp. 169–171.
3. Ibid, p. 149.

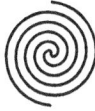

Acknowledgments

Thank you to Caitlin Harris for the glorious cover and Diane Rigoli for the brilliant design of the book. Thank you to Eberhardt Press and the IPRC for your help in bringing this project to life.

Thank you to Jennifer Ruby Privateer and Vanessa Veselka for your fabulous editing and to my first readers, Jane Meredith and Brandon Claycomb, for infinitely helpful suggestions. Thanks to my dear colleagues in the IPRC program and the leadership of Justin Hocking who reminded me that anything was possible.

Thank you to my teachers and initiators of this writing, teaching, body, soul and world healing craft—Elizabeth Checchio, Martha Gies, Vanessa Veselka, Lidia Yuknavitch, Lorie Dechar, Benjamin Fox, Sean Tuten, Starhawk, Nina Simons, Jen Louden, Joanna Macy, Stephen Levine

Thanks to Diana Fried, Carla Cassler and Melanie Rubin of Acupuncturists Without Borders who taught me that post-traumatic stress is not invincible and cycles of trauma in the world can be broken.

Thank you to all the luminary healers, artists and activists interviewed in ROS. Keep going. The vision you bring to this world is essential.

Thanks to my tireless agent, Nancy Ellis, for believing in this book.

Thanks to my Portland writing group: Ellen, Max, Julie, Robin, Peter, Jerry, and Myrla for your critique, advice and entertainment.

Thanks to my healing and spiritual communities with whom I have made art, ritual, theatre and magic for many years—Reclaiming,

Omnirootz, Enchanted Spiral, Common Ground Wellness Center, Feri, Acupuncturists Without Borders, Center for Healing and Rejuvenation, Source Material and more. You, my colleagues, are some of the most talented and wise global revolutionary healers in the world.

Thanks to my students, patients and clients for challenging me and allowing me the great honor to work beside you as a teacher and healer. You make me these things.

Thanks to my biological family for creating the most perfect scenarios to awaken the medicine in me. You made me a healer.

And all thanks to the most supportive family of friends for feeding me, holding me, standing up for me, forgiving me, inspiring me, pushing me, and telling me the truth during this process, especially Bri, Blaed, Charlie, Chris, CJ, Crow, Danny, Dawn, Diana, Fio, Jane Meredith, James, Jesse, Jim, Lilith, Linda, Lynx, Kelly, Madrone, Molly, Nikole, Nina, Ravenna, Rosie, Seraphina, Suzanne, Urania, Vanessa, and Willow. In the hardest times, your kind of love heals everything. I am so lucky.

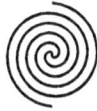

Author Biography

Gerri Ravyn Stanfield is a transformational acupuncturist and business coach, an inventive author, and international educator. She practices acupuncture in Portland, Oregon with a focus on helping people survive cancer, chronic pain and traumatic experiences. She uses her background in the realms of social justice, Taoist/Chinese medicine, Jungian psychology, Acupuncturists Without Borders, earth based religions, and creative writing to coax more of the extraordinary into the world through the cracks in Western civilization. She is dedicated to liberating the medicine within each of us.

Ravyn is a cultural alchemist, seeking to transform the heart-break of living in our modern world into gold. She creates theatre and ritual art, weaving poetry, music and performance into contemporary offerings of the human imagination. Many of her original songs show up in rituals and songbooks worldwide. She has developed in-person and online trainings for universities, non-profits and the Oregon prison system. She designs apprenticeship programs for emerging leaders and healers in various communities throughout the US, Canada, Europe, Asia and Australia and offers yearlong Sacred Leadership trainings. This is her first book.

www.gerriravynstanfield.com